GOOD GUT, GREAT HEALTH

THE FULL GUIDE TO OPTIMIZING YOUR ENERGY AND VITALITY

Vicki Edgson & Adam Palmer

Based on the health regime created by
Elaine Williams and Stephanie Moore
of Grayshott Spa

Photography by Lisa Linder

jacqui
small

First published in 2015 by
Jacqui Small LLP
74–77 White Lion Street
London N1 9PF

This paperback edition published 2017

Publisher: Jacqui Small
Senior Commissioning Editor: Fritha Saunders
Designer: Maggie Town
Editor: Heather Thomas
Photographer: Lisa Linder
Production: Maeve Healy

ISBN: 978 1 910254 92 9

A catalogue record for this book is
available from the British Library.

2019 2018 2017
10 9 8 7 6 5 4 3 2 1

Printed in China

Quarto is the authority on a wide range of topics.
Quarto educates, entertains and enriches the lives of our
readers — enthusiasts and lovers of hands-on living.

www.QuartoKnows.com

Key to recipe symbols:

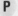 **P**   Plan recipes

P+   Post-Plan recipes

CONTENTS

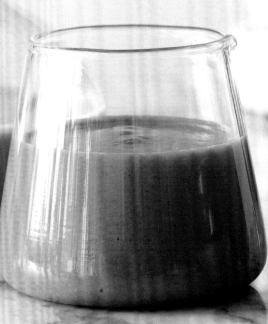

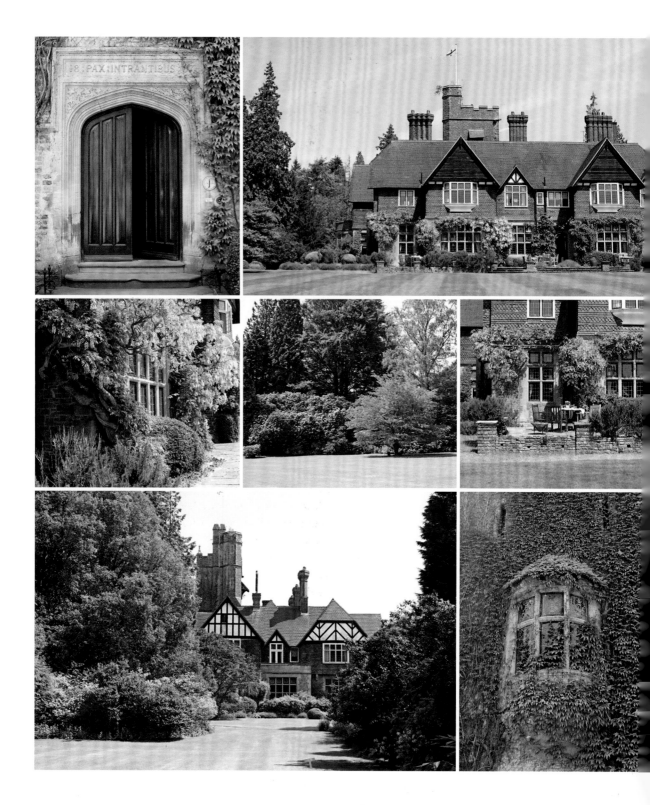

Foreword
by Simon Lowe
Owner and CEO, Grayshott Spa, Surrey, UK

Since Grayshott Hall became a spa 50 years ago, the medical profession, pharmaceutical and food industries – as well as people all over the world – have become increasingly concerned about their health, as manifested in their diet, level of fitness and personal appearance. Governments and the private sector have devoted vast resources to telling us what to eat, how to exercise and the dire consequences of not taking advice from the experts and corporations that bombard us daily with publications and advertisements offering remedies and potions that, allegedly, will help us to achieve healthier, fitter and more beautiful bodies.

I have observed the exaggerated claims of nirvana from diets with more and more scepticism. In most cases, what is on offer cannot and does not deliver sustainable results, especially as increasingly bizarre combinations of exotic foods, meal programmes and impossible timetables are devised. These are pushed to an ever-expanding audience that is desperate for success but inevitably disappointed by the reality of what they are being sold as well as their own inability to sustain the prescribed utopian solutions.

I believe that a more transparent, no-nonsense world would produce an audience receptive to the fact that most solutions offered are simply a waste of time and money. However, there are effective solutions and these are the ones that are produced by people whose expertise can deliver results with integrity.

I decided to gather my team at Grayshott and research and assemble a health programme that would address some of the symptoms and consequences of modern living. We believe that repairing 'the gut' is the key to restorative good health. As the godfather of medicine said: *'All diseases begin in the gut'.* Hippocrates (460 – 370 B.C.)

Through therapeutic treatments, herbal tinctures, a scientifically backed diet and specific eating practices, we believe that health must be tackled from the inside out, and the nutrition we recommend is based on a naturopathic approach to gut cleansing and rebalancing the digestive system. The crucial first step to vibrant health is often overlooked: understanding the delicate and complex processes of the digestive system.

At Grayshott we are fortunate to have a wonderful team who have come together to share their expertise, knowledge and experience. What is so exciting is that our programme has delivered results and, even more important, it is sustainable, which is the key to its success. Many readers may have visited clinics all over the world and emerged feeling wonderful only to relapse into their old routine, negating their efforts to achieve their goals because they could not maintain the prescribed diet or exercise regime.

Most of us want to feel healthy and good about ourselves. Although there is no universal panacea or cure for obesity, diabetes and the aches and pains of modern living, I believe that our approach not only works but is 'doable' and sustainable. Providing you can take something from it, it will help you achieve your goals and deliver lasting results.

The route to true health
by Elaine Williams and Stephanie Moore of Grayshott Spa

Nutrition has always been a cornerstone of our health philosophy at Grayshott Spa. Two years ago we pooled our collective 50 years of clinical research, experience and practice to develop a more structured programme for our guests and created The Grayshott Health Regime. One of the main factors influencing our approach was our concern about people's often misguided notions of needing to 'detoxify' and their desire for a spartan, punitive regime to achieve this. We felt this was mistaken as the demands of modern life, such as over-work, over-exercise, over-fatigue and continuous exposure to stress, were leaving people depleted and in need of nourishment rather than cleansing through deprivation. One of the main casualties of such a lifestyle is a compromised digestive system, and from this emerged the core of our Plan, which focuses on digestive health as the route to true health.

We not only wanted to show people how to regain good health and nourish their bodies through eating real food but also to make them understand that eating the appropriate foods would support and take care of detoxification. This enables us to confidently recommend eating delicious, healing and satisfying foods, such as good-quality, grass-fed red meats (including the fat), fish, eggs, fermented foods, butter, cream, nuts, avocado and a rainbow of wonderful, organic vegetables.

On the Plan, our guests have noticed improvements in their health in as little as one week. We knew that these principles worked over several weeks or months but never imagined the dramatic results that could be attained on such a focused programme. We have repeatedly recorded measureable improvement in such markers as blood glucose, serum cholesterol, triglycerides and gamma GT.

Whilst these objective health measurements have excited us and various members of the medical fraternity, our clients are more often thrilled with the unexpected weight loss aspect, especially as it is body fat that has been lost and not muscle. This reinforces our long-held conviction not to make weight loss the primary focus, as it will often take care of itself as the body heals. We regard being over or under weight as merely a sign of a deeper problem. Correct that and people generally achieve a healthy weight.

We hope readers of this book will enjoy undertaking this Plan as much as our guests at the spa. We are immensely grateful to Vicki Edgson for undertaking the arduous task of writing about it in order that it may reach a wider audience, and also to Adam Palmer for creating such delicious and nourishing recipes.

Enjoy your abundant health.

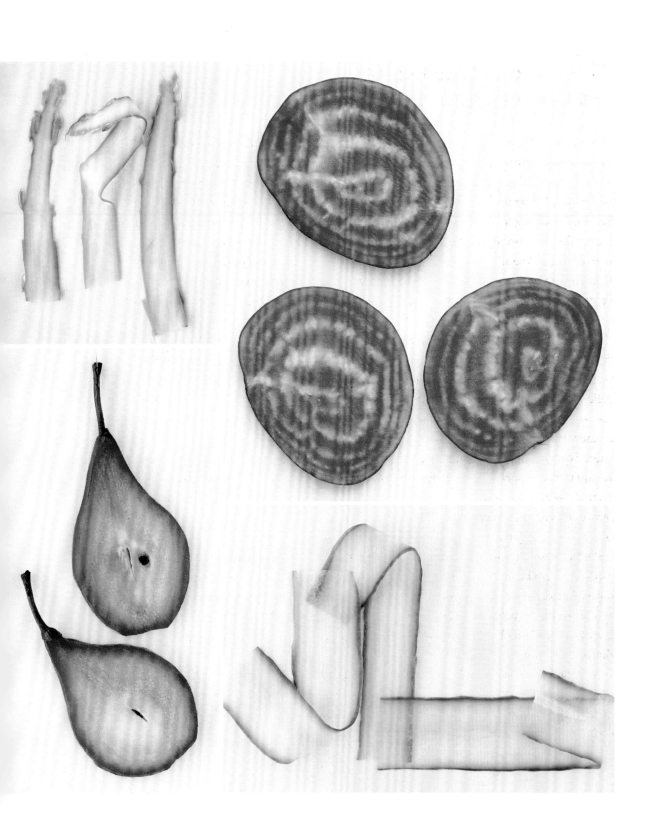

Introduction

The Good Gut, Great Health Plan is not a diet but a way of eating that has evolved over the last few years thanks to extensive research. It is based on sound naturopathic principles, updated with new knowledge, and it has been tried and tested on hundreds of people to determine how important it is to eat well – all the time. In a world that is increasingly questioning where its food is coming from, and how it is grown or reared, there's never been a more important time to take an interest in what you put into your mouth.

The principles of the Good Gut, Great Health Plan are listed opposite. These provide the outline of the Plan and encourage you to eat a broader range of healthy foods rather than just sticking to the daily staples that many of us tend to eat, day in, day out. The essence of the Plan is that your palate and digestion fare best when you consume a variety of foods that are seasonal and preferably grown locally and as close to home as possible.

This book teaches us that cleaning up the digestive system is the key to sustainable good health. Just in the same way that we clean our teeth and wash our hair on a regular basis, so should we look after our digestive system. It is part of the parasympathetic nervous system, which means that, like breathing and heartbeat, it's one of the parts of the body that functions 24:7. However, it has now been proven that refraining from eating periodically – known as intermittent fasting – gives the digestive system time to heal and repair itself as well as other long-term benefits. When practised over a number of months, intermittent fasting helps to naturally lower blood pressure as well as damaging LDL (low-density lipoprotein) cholesterol, and restore balance.

You can achieve this on the Plan by choosing two days a week (separate, not concurrent, days) on which you limit your food intake. You can have one bowl of chicken or beef stock, which has been simmered for several hours to extract the most dense amount of nutrients out of the carcass or bones. This is the last dish you eat before going to bed one evening until lunchtime the following day. This 'cleansing' is more than manageable – it is positively energizing, as digestion uses up a lot of energy and giving it a break allows this energy to be used elsewhere in the body.

The Plan yields enormous benefits, as has been seen repeatedly at Grayshott Spa where it has been offered to hundreds of guests with amazing results. Read the following pages to discover its benefits as well as how you can put it into practice on a daily basis; then try the delicious recipes, which are highly nutritious and embody the principles of the Plan (see opposite).

The 10 principles of the Plan

1 Although it's still a science in its infancy we know that digestive health is dependent on healthy gut bacteria, with as much as 85 per cent of immunity affected by it. Creating healthy gut flora is at the heart of the Plan.

2 Eating fermented foods regularly is integral to sustaining healthy gut bacteria. The Plan focuses on fermented vegetables, which are packed with healthy probiotics and prebiotics (non-digestible fibre).

3 On the Plan we eliminate grains, most pulses and some vegetables, depending on their molecular structure and how they are physiologically broken down. This is why dairy is omitted – the lactose molecule is too complex for a resting digestive system.

4 We encourage you to eat healthy fats every day for nourishment and their anti-inflammatory properties.

5 Good-quality protein is essential at each meal, with animal proteins preferable to vegetable ones, as they are easier for the body to break down and utilize.

6 Meats should preferably be from organic, grass-fed livestock, which is high in anti-inflammatory Omega-3 fatty acids and less likely to contain antibiotics that are detrimental to beneficial micro-organisms in the gut.

7 Fruit and vegetables should be organic where possible to avoid the antibacterial sprays and pesticides that are so harmful to the gut.

8 Always blanch vegetables for eating in salads. The blanching partially deconstructs the cellulose structure and makes it easier for the gut to extract the nutrients.

9 Ensure that all the permitted nuts, seeds and pulses are soaked for 24 hours prior to cooking. This eliminates enzyme inhibitors that can weaken the digestive function.

10 Avoid alcohol while you are on the Plan as this is an anti-inflammatory programme and alcohol affects inflammation in the same way that pouring petrol onto flames affects a fire.

How your body works

It is now understood, as well as being a well-accepted fact in medical and complementary therapy circles, that most disease begins in the gut – as Hippocrates famously said, 'let food be your medicine, and medicine be your food'. The *Good Gut, Great Health* approach appreciates the function of the entire digestive system, from mouth to bowel, and what you need to do physically and emotionally to improve and optimize it. On the opposite page, you can see how the digestive system works, and its total interaction from top to bottom as the food you eat travels through your body. Digestion must be efficient in the stomach in order for the rest of the system to function optimally, and this is why we suggest 'eating mindfully'.

Eating mindfully

Choosing fresh food carefully, and paying attention to where it is sourced, is as important as balancing proteins and carbohydrates, as set out in this Plan. Much of the food we eat is now mass-produced and bought in supermarkets, paying little respect to its seasonal availability or where it is grown or reared. We recommend that you visit your local farmers' markets to find out which foods grow best at different times of the year, and buy produce that has been sun-ripened and grown or raised with ethical and humane resources. Grass-fed animals are more relaxed and less stressed than their mass-farmed counterparts, and this is transmitted into the food itself. Intensively-farmed chickens producing eggs at twice their natural speed yield less healthy ones than free-range hens, as their nutrients have not had enough time to mature.

THINK ABOUT WHAT YOU ARE EATING

The recipes in this book encourage you to eat more mindfully. Make time to prepare fresh food (sometimes ahead of when you actually eat it if it's practical to do so) that nourishes your body and satisfies your appetite. Think carefully about how much sugar is added to processed food – it interferes with the pancreatic release of insulin, leading to cravings for more of the same. Eating a balance of fresh foods (the permitted proteins, carbohydrates and fats) provides the nutrients you need without having to resort to sugar for energy.

Eating mindfully means you need to set aside a suitable time and a relaxing environment in which to eat. Focus on what you are eating rather than combining two or three tasks simultaneously. Always chew your food carefully and consider how nourishing it is. Learn to recognize when you have eaten enough and do not eat more than you need, even if some food is left on your plate – it's not wasteful to leave it if you feel full. Your stomach will let your brain know when it's had sufficient food. This 'training' of brain-to-stomach communication occurs naturally and you simply have to recognize it and stop eating when you've had enough.

WHAT YOU SHOULD EAT

Over the following pages, we will address the specific foods, flavourings, herbs and spices that have a beneficial effect on your digestive system as a whole. The increasing incidence of disease and obesity in Western societies illustrates how detrimental processed and highly-sweetened foods are for your digestion and, subsequently, your health. You need to eat carbohydrates, proteins and fats to nourish your mind and body and have a healthy digestive system that absorbs and eliminates foods efficiently. We highlight the foods that you should avoid eating, and why, so you can recognize which ones are healthy and best to eat. However, first you need to understand how the digestive system works, as this is the crux of the Plan – this is explained in the flow chart opposite.

How the digestive system works

The mouth is where digestion begins, with the production of ptyalin, a digestive enzyme that is secreted from the first thought, smell or sight of food. Chewing your food thoroughly is vital for proper digestion. By the time your first mouthful hits the stomach, it should have been broken down into a form resembling a thick liquid.

The stomach works like a washing machine via the various sets of muscles that turn, churn and break down the food even more to ensure that the components can be absorbed in the small and large intestines. The stomach has the only highly acid environment of the digestive tract, with a variable pH (the measurement of variability of acidity or alkalinity) of 1.2–4.5, providing it is secreting sufficient hydrochloric acid and proteases (enzymes that break down the highly-dense proteins we need to eat on this Plan). This acidity also ensures that any damaging bacteria that may reside in the food is neutralized and killed off.

The pancreas performs two functions:
1 **Digestive**: releasing the digestive enzyme, protease (for proteins); amylase (for carbohydrates); and lipase (for fats) to aid digestion in the small intestine.
2 **Producing hormones**: insulin, to help regulate your blood sugar levels and let you know when you are full by transporting glucose (the end product of digestion) to the brain and muscles for energy; and leptin, to tell your brain when you are full. These hormones work in tandem, telling your brain when you have had sufficient nutrients to satisfy your body and brain.

The liver produces bile salts that join with bile from the gall bladder, together emulsifying or breaking down fats from the food we eat. Eating the right kind of fat feeds the body with nutrient-dense compounds that are vital for the brain and nervous system to function well and produce the hormones we need.

The small intestine is the first part of the digestive system that actually absorbs the essential nutrients derived from the combination of mono-saccharide carbohydrates – the simplest form of carbohydrates, which are the vegetables and fruits that are the easiest to digest (see pages 24–28) – with proteins from animal sources (meats, poultry and dairy), and essential fats found in fish, nuts and seeds. Ninety per cent of all foodstuffs are absorbed through the small intestine, where billions of finger-like projections, called villi, increase the total absorption area of the gut lining.

The large intestine's health is dependent on all the digestive functions working correctly, as well as good peristalsis (muscular movement that pushes the faecal matter through the large intestine for elimination) to prevent constipation. Absorption of any remaining nutrients (10 per cent) occurs here, but you need to include sufficient fibre in your diet to ensure regular movement and prevent the waste matter being reabsorbed through the intestinal wall.

How stress affects digestion

Stress in the body comes in many forms, and it is not simply emotional. It precipitates a hormonal cascade of responses and it can be caused by:

Consumed substances: prescribed and/or recreational drugs, alcohol, excess caffeine, sugars and sweeteners, processed foods, flavour-enhancers, artificial colourings and fungicides, pesticides and growth-enhancers in food.
Heavy metals: mercury and amalgam fillings in teeth, pins in joints, and body-piercing.
Environmental elements: pollution, poor air supply, air-conditioning, air travel, IT exposure, dehydration.
Emotional factors: divorce, the loss of a loved one, redundancy, post-natal stress, anger, hurt, resentment, fear, intimidation and bullying; financial worries, debt.

High cortisol levels (produced by the adrenal glands in times of stress) will inhibit both the digestive function and how full you feel after eating. Cortisol, the hormone that is released in response to a stressor to the body or mind, is a primordial reaction to the 'fight or flight' syndrome in the early days of man.

In those days, there would have been surges of cortisol release as a man hunted, allowing him to run faster and further with heightened awareness and response mechanisms that would either save his life or provide his next meal. There would then follow a period when the release of cortisol would abate and early man would relax, eat and sleep to give his muscles time to recover. Cortisol is important for survival, instigating every movement and motivating our brains, but it should be produced on an on-off basis.

Feeding the brain

As much as 80 per cent of what we eat is used to feed the brain, before the remainder of the body's organs are nourished, so a 'foggy brain' or 'feeling fatigued,' often indicates that we need to eat more fresh, nutrient-dense food. Once you have followed this programme for at least 21 days, you will start to feel more mentally alert as well as more energetic physically.

Nowadays, the cortisol-release response is often in a permanently 'switched-on' mode. Our adrenal glands (found above the kidneys), which secrete cortisol, become over-worked and under-nourished, especially when caffeine and 'quick-fix' foods and drinks are used to keep going rather than listening to our body and mind when they are exhausted. This state can lead to increased blood pressure, heart disease, anxiety and panic attacks. This type of stress in the body can also be a contributory factor in inflammatory conditions, especially in the gut, where bloating, wind, constipation, pain and discomfort may become the norm for many people. Learning to eat slowly and mindfully (see page 12) will help to abate such problems considerably, allowing the digestion to function optimally.

Why antioxidants are so important

Antioxidant nutrients protect us against cellular damage, through wear and tear, through the body's natural metabolic processes and the effects of stress (in any form). They also prevent premature ageing in our skin, brain, heart, vitality and energy. The antioxidant vitamins and minerals (opposite) are found in many brightly coloured foods, especially the vegetables and berry fruits on the Plan. These are phytonutrients ('phyto' means plant-based); ideally, they should be organic so the salvestrols (anti-cancer and anti-ageing compounds) found in the skins of many of them are not contaminated. Salvestrols are recognized for their ability to help neutralize cancer cells without harming the surrounding healthy cells. Animal proteins provide abundant antioxidant zinc and selenium – vital for protecting organs, such as the thyroid, liver and skin.

Vegetable sources of proteins, found in nuts, seeds and their oils as well as lentils, are also good but do not contain all nine essential amino acids like their animal counterparts. However, they do contain both vitamins and minerals, unlike animal proteins, which are much higher in minerals. Antioxidants work together to support and protect us and they are more powerful this way. Many of the foods you can eat on the Plan contain the main antioxidant nutrients within them.

The main antioxidants

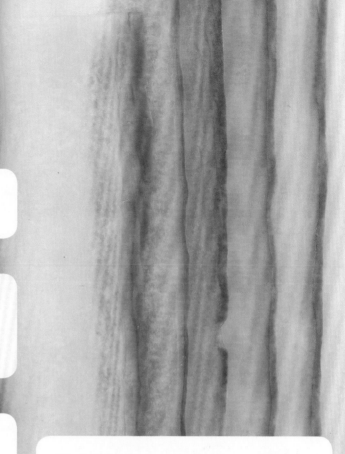

Vitamin A (animal-based): found in beef, lamb, calves' liver and kidneys.

Beta-carotene (vegetable-based form of vitamin A): found in cherries, berries (all), carrots, beetroot (beets), red cabbage, aubergine (eggplant), red and orange tomatoes.

Vitamin C: in bell peppers, kiwi, broccoli, kale, chard, spinach, peas, tomatoes, citrus fruits and papaya

Glutathione (known as the master antioxidant, recharging all the other antioxidants): found in avocado, asparagus, onions, garlic, spinach, broccoli and green leafy vegetables, apples, turmeric, red meat, chicken, eggs and fermented dairy (post-Plan only).

Vitamin E: found in avocado, sesame seeds, chia, sunflower and pumpkin seeds, all nuts and their oils.

Selenium: in shrimps, sardines, salmon, scallops, cod, chicken, turkey, lamb, beef, cashews, macadamia nuts, walnuts, Brazil nuts, sunflower and pumpkin seeds.

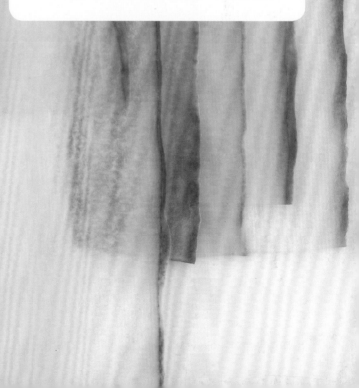

Zinc: found in shellfish, including oysters, mussels and shrimps, eggs, beef, lamb, venison, chicken, duck, pecans, walnuts, almonds, mushrooms and cocoa.

Know what you're eating

In this section we explain the 10 Good Gut, Great Health principles in greater detail, so that you can better understand the foundations of the Plan. We recommend you follow the Plan for at least three weeks to ensure the restorative health of your digestive system. This may start immediately, but it takes from seven to twenty-one days for some people to experience tangible and noticeable results. A 14-day meal-planner is provided on page 49 to suggest how you can get the right balance of the different food groups. Post-Plan eating is explained in Taking it Further (see page 50), illustrating which foods can be re-introduced to promote intestinal health.

The Plan – making the change

Like many people, you may be unaware that you have digestive problems, but following this Plan will help normalize your weight, improve your skin, hair and nails, and benefit the way your brain functions, helping you to think more clearly. A well-functioning digestive system is fundamental to the nutrient absorption you require for optimal health. Once you realize how healthy it's possible to feel on the Plan, you are also less likely to revert to your pre-Plan habits.

A considered caution

People with more serious digestive conditions, such as irritable bowel syndrome, colitis or diverticulitis, should follow the Plan until all of their symptoms have abated rather than moving on too quickly to the post-Plan.

BOOSTING YOUR DIGESTIVE JUICES

On the Plan, we recommend you eat 2 teaspoons of sauerkraut or other fermented foods just before every main meal to stimulate stomach acid and enzyme production. You can do this by consuming digestive bitters, home-made sauerkrauts and foods such as preserved pickled mushrooms (see page 151). They help to trigger bile production and pancreatic function.

HYDRATION

Hydration is key to a well-functioning gut in addition to being essential for almost all physiological processes. The best way to hydrate your body is to drink plenty of still filtered water with a slice of lemon added or whichever herbal teas you like. Avoid drinking fruit juices, alcohol and caffeinated drinks, such as tea and coffee, on the Plan, as these are all severely disruptive to the ecology of the gut lining.

INTERMITTENT FASTING

We now know a considerable amount about the benefits of intermittent (partial) fasting, a practice that has been around for thousands of years across many cultures. On the Plan we recommend that you follow the intermittent fasting outlined in the 14-day meal planner section (see page 49), to allow the gut to rest, encourage cellular renewal and reduce the speed of the ageing process. The benefits of reducing your intake of food periodically have been well-researched and documented extensively.

If you do it on an ongoing basis, intermittent fasting can reduce damaging LDL cholesterol, lower blood pressure that may have been too high, and re-balance blood sugar levels (reducing the potential for developing type 2 diabetes). It can also be useful if you have problems maintaining a healthy weight and can help to reduce weight gain around the middle of the body. If you want to enjoy excellent general health and give your gut a rest occasionally, we further recommend that you make intermittent fasting part of your lifestyle rather than considering it as dieting. Other long-term benefits include improved sleep patterns and increased focus and attention as you give your gut the opportunity to heal and repair itself on a regular basis.

Foods to enjoy on the Plan

Organic and grass-fed livestock (meats, poultry and game, eggs) should be chosen if possible to prevent consuming hormones or inappropriate cattle-feed. This guarantees a better-quality diet and more satisfying food, without stressing your body unduly. These form the majority of the essential proteins for healing and repair. The ratio of Omega-3:-6 is higher in grass-fed livestock, making this a healthier choice.

Deep-water fish feed on krill and other microscopic sea-borne foods that increase their Omega-3, which is both anti-inflammatory and nourishing to the brain and the entire nervous system. Oily fish (sardines, mackerel, etc.) should be consumed at least three times per week on the Plan as it is another excellent source of protein. Eat naturally-smoked fish (available from most supermarkets) to avoid the chemicals found in commercially-smoked varieties.

Fruits, vegetables and salad leaves should be eaten in season, so they are naturally ripened rather than having been shipped from the other side of the world. Seasonal foods, which are locally sourced and ripened to their full capacity, are easy to digest as their inherent enzymes create healthy digestive support. They are essential for their fibre and antioxidants.

Lentils, butter (lima) beans and split peas should always be soaked and well-cooked to reduce the enzyme inhibitors and make them easier to digest. Avoid all other pulses and legumes while you are on the Plan.

Foods to avoid on the Plan

Dairy foods You should not consume cow's, goat's or sheep's milk, cheese or yoghurt while you are on the Plan. Some people are lactose-intolerant, which interferes with the normal functioning of the gut, creating inflammation. We also omit soy milk as many of the commercially-available sources may be derived from genetically-modified soya beans, which can be hormone-disruptive. Nut milks, made from soaked almonds, hazelnuts and cashews, are viable alternatives, as is coconut milk. They all contain good levels of protein, essential fats and minerals that are calming to the digestive system.

Grains All grains are prohibited on the Plan as they are complex carbohydrates, causing disruption and inflammation to intestinal cells and interfering with the function of the villi (the microscopic finger-like projections in the lining of the intestines that greatly increase the total surface area of absorption of the nutrients in food). Grains are also far too complex in structure and need greater digestion to break them down, interfering with the rest and repair of the gut.

Alcohol Avoid drinking any alcohol while you're on the Plan. It has the potential to inflame the gut lining and disrupt blood sugar levels, causing subsequent highs and lows in mood and energy levels. All alcohol contains a certain amount of sugars used in the fermentation process. Organic and fermented biodynamic red wines are high in antioxidants, and you can have these occasionally post-Plan but only with food.

The food groups

Getting the right balance of proteins, carbohydrates and beneficial fats is essential if you want to feel better and healthier. Many diets exclude one of these three food groups in order to force the body to use stored fat for fuel. However, this is neither a sustainable nor a healthy approach, as foods from all the various food groups are needed to perform different functions in the body. Whilst there are certain restrictions on the Plan that are designed to allow the gut to heal, there is never a shortage of food from all three groups.

Perfect proteins

Protein – both animal and vegetable – is vital for rebuilding and repairing all the cells in the body. The word is taken from the Greek word *protos*, meaning 'first things', and every part of the development of a foetus is dependent on it. Proteins are the essence of the Plan, helping to balance blood sugar levels, preventing cravings and assisting in regulating the hormone leptin, which is produced in the fat cells and tells the hypothalamus in the brain to let us know when we are full. In the large intestine, the amino acids from the proteins we eat are an essential component for repairing the intestinal villi, through which we absorb essential nutrients from our food.

It is far easier to get the nutrients we need from animal-based proteins than vegetable-sourced ones, especially if your digestive system is weak. They are in a much simpler form to digest and absorb, and magnesium, B12 and iron (important for cardiovascular health, hormone balance and digestive function) from animal produce are easier for the body to use.

HOW MUCH PROTEIN DO WE NEED?

We are only able to obtain the nine essential amino acids (histidine, leucine, lysine, isoleucine, methionine, phenylalanine, threonine, valine and tryptophan) from the foods we eat as we are unable to manufacture them in the body. All nine of them are found in animal proteins, whereas the vegetable alternatives (nuts and seeds, some pulses and beans, grains and their derivatives, such as tahini spread made from sesame seed and olive oil) contain only some of the nine amino acids, and therefore they need to be eaten together to provide all the essential components. This is one of the reasons why the animal protein element of the Plan is so important, with organic eggs and grass-fed livestock being such a vital part of what you can eat.

Protein takes far longer than carbohydrates for the body to digest, break down and absorb, which helps to regulate the rate at which insulin is released and prevents an abrupt rise in blood sugar levels, reducing the risk of developing diabetes. Adults need approximately 25–30g(1oz) of protein per meal in order to support healthy fitness, re-growth and repair of the body. These can come from a combination of both animal and vegetable proteins, so you don't need to eat only animal-sourced ones. For instance, ful medames for breakfast (see page 73) will provide a combination of both animal- (eggs) and vegetable-based (lentils) proteins. However, we recommend that you include some animal protein in your evening meal on the days when you're not fasting to prevent hunger cravings and also to make sure that your sleep is not interrupted by roller-coaster blood sugar levels.

A QUESTION OF ORGANICS?

All animal proteins should be organic and grass-fed where possible, to avoid the growth hormones, antibiotics and mass-farming methods that are employed worldwide. Some of these animals are fed with grains that are possibly unsuitable for their own

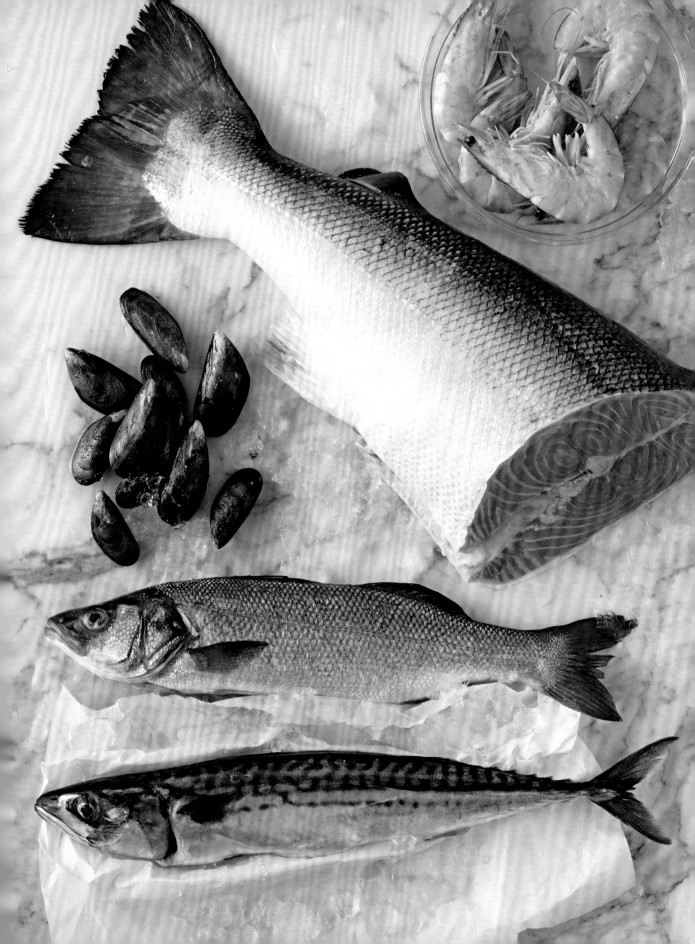

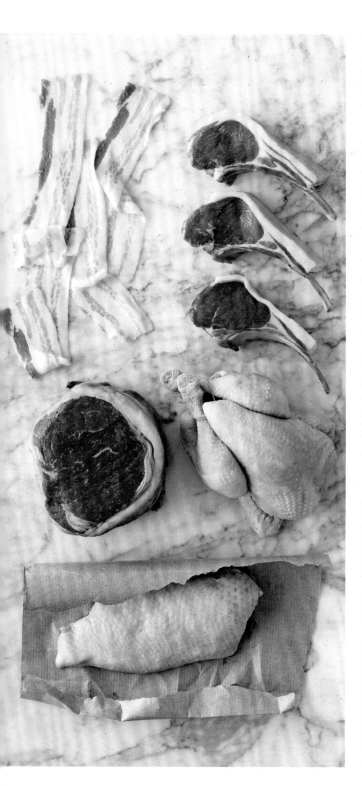

digestive systems, leading to distress and stresses that are reflected in the produce they yield. This is particularly important for cattle and chickens that have been farmed inhumanely and may be riddled with antibiotics to combat a range of diseases.

All the produce we recommend should be organic, especially eggs, which feature in many of the recipes on this Plan, as they contain all the nutrients required for your body and brain, as well as providing a relatively low-cost, nutrient-dense food that is versatile, suitable for all the family, and may be eaten on a daily basis in one form or another.

When it comes to fish, the question of whether or not you should purchase 'wild' or 'farmed' is more complex, as most available fish is now farmed to some extent, so we recommend that you opt only for 'sustainably farmed', as these farms have to take more care over the development and nourishment of their produce.

All the fish that is now sold in the Western world in supermarkets or served in restaurants has been flash-frozen on catching by law, as the boats that fish on this scale are often at sea for several days. This actually preserves the fish in its freshest state and ensures that it reaches the packing distributors in as close to a 'just caught' state as is possible. It is only when you have

Why avoid dairy produce?

The casein portion (protein) of animal dairy produce can be inflammatory and mucus-forming, irritating the absorptive cells (enterocytes) in the intestinal lining, and interfering with the integrity of the gut and the absorption of nutrients from the gut into the bloodstream. In some people, this can present as a genuine allergy, with severe abdominal cramps and diarrhoea (possible triggers for Crohn's disease and irritable bowel syndrome), whilst for most it is more of an intolerant reaction (lactose intolerance), such as runny nose, blocked sinuses or eczema. However mild the reaction, this is a constant challenge to the immune system, increasing the likelihood of sensitivity to other foods.

We recommend that you cut out all animal dairy produce, i.e. milk, cheese, cream, yoghurt, ice-cream and frozen yoghurt, for at least three weeks whilke you're on the Plan.

ANIMAL-BASED PROTEINS AT-A-GLANCE

PLAN PROTEIN	NUTRIENTS	GOOD FOR
MEAT Lamb, beef, pork, pancetta, ham, venison	Iron, calcium, zinc, all B vitamins, vitamin E, CLA (conjugated linoleic acid), Omega-3 and -6 essential fats.	Bone health, energy, low-GI, encouraging balanced blood sugar levels, weight loss, strengthening hair, nails and skin, supporting immunity, anti-inflammatory.
OFFAL Calves' liver, chicken liver, kidneys	High vitamin A, all B vitamins, and D, iron, zinc, copper, Omega-3 and -6 essential fats.	Bone health, cardiovascular strength, benefiting hair, skin and nails, boosting immunity.
POULTRY Duck, chicken, turkey, guinea fowl, quail, pheasant	Zinc, phosphorus, B vitamins, Omega-3 and -6 essential fats.	Boosting immunity, natural antibiotic properties, boosting metabolism and energy production, good skin, hair and nails.
EGGS All varieties of eggs are permitted	Perfect protein, vitamins A, D, E, all B vitamins, calcium, iron and manganese.	Brain, bone and ligament strength, hair, teeth and nails, boosting immunity, first-class protein.
OILY FISH (NOT SMOKED) Salmon, sardines, mackerel	Omega-3, vitamin E, calcium, phosphorus, selenium and iodine.	Boosting immunity, strengthening and hydrating all cells, bones, skin and hair, brain, nervous system, memory.
WHITE FISH Halibut, turbot, cod, haddock, sea bass, sea bream, lemon sole, Dover sole, mullet	Zinc and selenium, calcium, vitamin E, Omega-3 essential fats, folate and iodine.	Lean, low-GI energy, balancing blood sugar levels, supporting thyroid function, skin and hair, brain and cognitive function.
SHELLFISH Scallops, prawns, shrimps, squid, mussels, clams, crab	Highest source of zinc and selenium, iron, copper and B12.	Immunity, metabolism, energy, balancing blood sugar levels.

AVOID all dairy foods (except butter) and any processed meats, as well as meat and fish that are smoked using chemicals, and canned tuna.

bought fish from a fisherman on the dockside or in local fish markets that you know it has been caught that day. To choose the freshest fish is simple – the eyes should still be bright and not sunken, and the flesh should be very sweet and not at all fishy in odour or taste.

ANIMAL PROTEINS THAT ARE NOT ALLOWED

Not all animal proteins are good for you – on the Plan, make sure you avoid the following:

• **Canned fish:** this should never be eaten unless the fish has been preserved in brine – and the can is lined with a non-aluminum inner lining. Also, avoid canned fish that comes in a tomato-based sauce, as the acidity of the tomatoes carry the aluminum into the fish, which can

damage the neurological system. Always make sure that you rinse all canned fish thoroughly, and pat it dry with absorbent kitchen paper before adding it to salads, pâtés or other dishes.

• **Tuna:** all tuna, fresh and canned, contains mercury residues and aluminum in its fatty tissues. Don't eat it. This is particularly important if you are pregnant.

• **Smoked or processed meats:** with the exception of genuine oak-smoked meats and fish, no processed meats should be eaten on this Plan, as they contain an array of additives and preservatives to prolong their shelf life and prevent discolouring. Choose deli produce over vacuum-wrapped alternatives for ensured freshness and minimum preservatives.

Vegetable-based proteins

Unlike animal-based proteins, vegetable proteins also contain an element of carbohydrate, which is why some of them are limited on the Plan. This is due to the ratio of protein:carbohydrate they contain and whether or not they are predominantly mono-saccharide, and therefore easier for the digestive system to break down without causing potential inflammation and gas.

LIMA AND HARICOT BEANS

These are the only two beans permitted in the first phase of the Plan (owing to their mono-saccharide carbohydrate content). Ideally, use dried beans and soak them in water with a little lemon juice added overnight before boiling them twice. If time doesn't allow for this, you may buy organic canned pulses for the post-Plan phase (see page 52) when any digestive problems have ceased. Always rinse them at least twice, as they contain a lot of salt and/or sugars to preserve them.

LENTILS AND SPLIT PEAS, ALL NUTS AND SEEDS, AND THEIR OILS

All lentils (Puy, green, brown, split red or yellow), split peas, nuts and seeds should be soaked in water for at least 12 hours before cooking in order to remove substances called phytates that are found just under their skins. These can irritate the gut, interfere with absorption of minerals and are very hard to digest.

Chia seeds and pumpkin, sunflower and sesame seeds should all be treated in the same way, but they may need less time to 'plump up' or hydrate. We suggest that you use this method both during the Plan and post-Plan, as many people do not realise how indigestible the coatings and skins of nuts and seeds can be.

Always be sure to rinse nuts and seeds well after soaking them to make sure that the phytates have been thoroughly removed. You can then dry them on absorbent kitchen paper, or place them on a baking tray at the lowest temperature in a preheated oven for 10–20 minutes to dry them out.

VEGETABLE-BASED PROTEINS AT-A-GLANCE

PLAN PROTEIN	NUTRIENTS	GOOD FOR
BEANS & PULSES Puy lentils, brown lentils, orange lentils, yellow and green split peas, haricot beans, lima beans	Calcium, magnesium, zinc, vitamins A, C and B vitamins. Twice the protein content of wheat or rice. Slow-release energy.	Lowering cholesterol, lowering blood pressure, balancing blood sugar levels, feeling full, weight loss.
NUTS Pistachios, hazelnuts, walnuts, pecans, Brazils, almonds, pine, peanuts, cashews, chestnuts (avoid chestnut flour) coconut (and its oil, flour, butter, water and milk)	Omega-3 and -6, calcium, vitamin E, oleic essential fat and managanese.	Lowering LDL cholesterol, heart health, hair, skin and nails, bone density, immunity, balancing blood sugar levels and cognitive function.
SEEDS Pumpkin, sunflower, sesame, Chia, alfalfa sprouts	Vitamin E, Omega-3 and -6 essential fats, zinc, selenium, calcium and manganese.	Heart health, lowering bad LDL cholesterol, regulating blood sugar, cognitive function.

AVOID toasted, roasted, flavoured varieties of nuts and seeds, as these are often heated too high, turning the essential fats rancid.

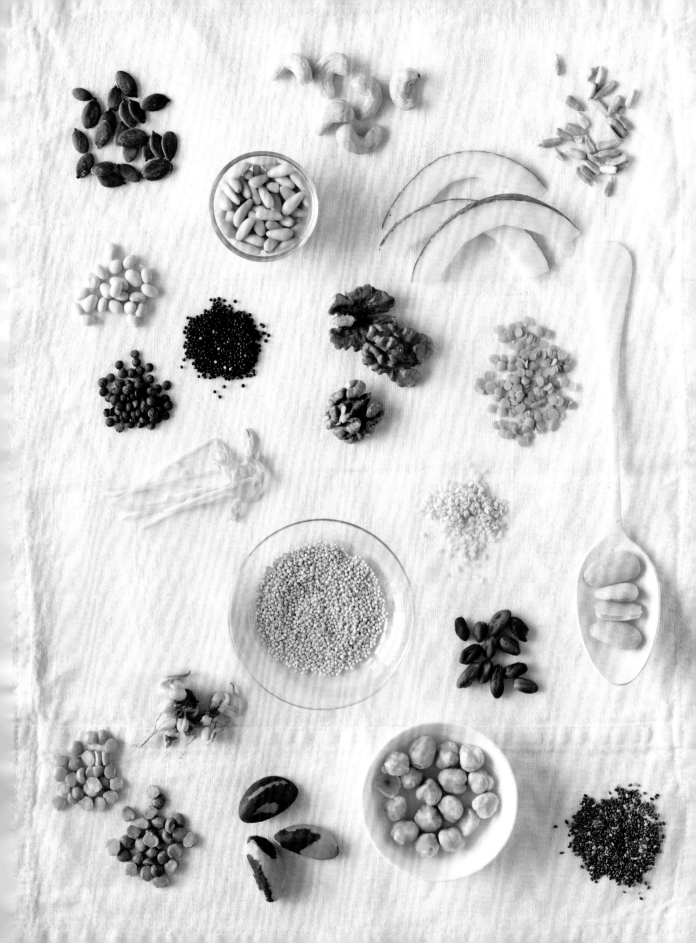

Carbohydrates

Carbohydrates account for many of the foods we eat and include all the grains, fruit and vegetables, as well as pulses, beans and peas (these also contain some proteins but they are not as complete in their amino-acid profile as animal-based protein). For many of us, carbohydrates provide the most abundant source of energy we need as fuel for our bodies. In this section we look at fruit and vegetables, as grains and pulses have already been covered in the previous pages under Proteins.

PERMITTED CARBOHYDRATES

Fruit and vegetables fall into sub-groups: the ones that can be broken down more readily into monosaccharides are the easiest to assimilate. Monosaccharides are carbohydrates in their simplest form; they enable the digestive system to absorb more of the nutrients it needs. Disaccharide (composed of two monosaccharides) or polysaccharide (long chains of monosaccharides) carbohydrates include potatoes, corn, sweet potatoes, parsnips and celeriac, as well as all sugars and sugar alternatives. Avoid these while you are on the Plan.

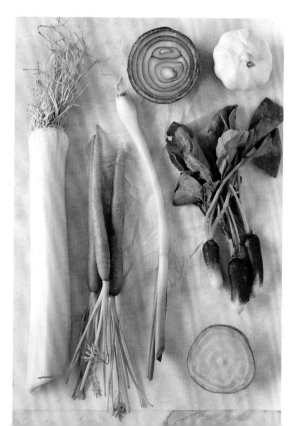

SAY 'NO' TO REFINED SUGARS AND CARBOHYDRATES

Cutting out all grains is a core part of the Plan as they are complex carbohydrates, which makes them too difficult for the resting gut to break down. This also includes the 'pseudo' grains, such as buckwheat, which are not strictly grains at all but behave in the gut in the same way. You can re-introduce these, along with other grains, including amaranth and basmati rice, post-Plan (see pages 50–53).

You should stop eating refined grains, which make up many of the cereals, biscuits, cakes, croissants and pastries that form a high percentage of our daily Western diet. Many of them contain sugar, preservatives and sweeteners, and they have had all their goodness ground, bleached and processed out of them, leaving very little in the way of worthwhile nutrients. These foods are the most damaging to the gut lining, along with alcohol and caffeine, as the sugars feed the damaging bacteria that cause bacterial infections in the body and kill off the beneficial bacteria that we need for a healthy gut (see page 13).

VEGETABLES

The root vegetables provide slow-release energy and antioxidants whereas green and leafy vegetables and salad leaves are packed with antioxidant protection, fibre and minerals that are essential for all the systems in the body. Eating a variety of vegetables is the key to promoting good health: each individual vegetable offers you a selection of nutrients, but when they are eaten collectively the choice is much broader and more comprehensive.

You need calcium and magnesium for contracting and relaxing muscles (including the heart) – these are found in many vegetables. The firmer the vegetable, the greater the calcium:magnesium ratio. Magnesium is important for the movement of the large intestine (peristalsis), whereas calcium is needed for a healthy nervous system, bones and teeth and blood clotting. This is why you need to eat a range of different vegetables every day.

We encourage you to eat an array of vegetables because of their fibre content, but also because on the Plan they are particularly important for their antioxidant capacity in healing and repairing the gut. Always choose seasonal vegetables and vary them as much as possible, preferably in a rainbow of colours, to make sure that you obtain a balance of all the nutrients they contain.

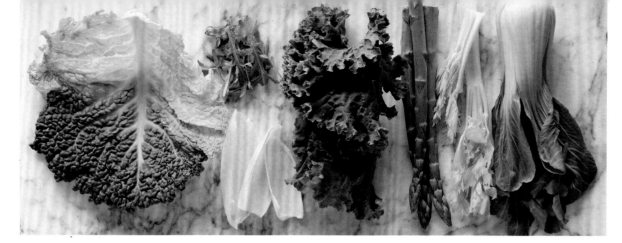

GREEN VEGETABLES AND SALAD LEAVES AT-A-GLANCE

VARIETY	NUTRIENTS	GOOD FOR
Artichokes	Vitamins C, K, folic acid, magnesium, manganese.	Diuretic properties, aiding digestion, improving stomach acidity, relieving IBS symptoms, detoxifying the liver, boosting gall bladder function, improving bile flow, stabilizing blood sugar.
Asparagus	Vitamins C, K, folic acid, manganese, potassium.	Energy, stimulating kidneys, antibacterial.
Bok choy	Vitamins A, C and K.	Healthy muscle and nerve function, immunity, antioxidant.
Broccoli	Vitamins A, C, K, potassium.	Intestinal cleanser, detoxifying, stimulating liver.
Cauliflower	Vitamins C, K, folic acid, manganese.	Purifying blood, bleeding gums, kidney and bladder disorders, high blood pressure and constipation, antioxidant.
Celery	Vitamins C, K, folic acid, potassium.	Lowering blood pressure, cardiovascular health, migraines, aiding digestion, arthritic joints.
Chard	Vitamins C, K, beta-carotene.	Eye protection, regulating blood sugar levels, bone health.
Courgette (zucchini)	Vitamin C, potassium.	Blood pressure, boosting immunity, stabilizing blood sugar and insulin levels, preventing constipation, relieving irritable bowel symptoms.
Cucumber	Vitamin C, potassium.	Helping absorption of iron, diuretic, laxative, helping digestion and regulating blood pressure.
Endive	Vitamins A, K, folic acid.	Asthma, anaemia, liver and gallbladder, weight loss.
Kale	Vitamin K, beta-carotene, iron, calcium.	Lowering cholesterol, antioxidant, eye health.
Lettuce	Vitamin K, beta-carotene, manganese.	Hydration, bones, joints, arteries and connective tissues.
Rocket (arugula)	Vitamins A, C, beta-carotene, calcium, folate, phytonutrients.	Liver health, bone health, eye and skin conditions.
Savoy cabbage	Vitamins B6, C and K, manganese.	Stimulating the immune system, killing bacteria and viruses, antioxidant, eaten raw – improving digestion and detoxifying stomach.
Spinach	Vitamin K, beta-carotene, manganese, magnesium.	Regulating blood pressure, boosting immune system, bone health, rich in antioxidants.
Watercress	Vitamins A, C, and K, calcium, iron.	Diuretic, breaking up kidney or bladder stones, purifying blood, stimulating thyroid.

ROOT VEGETABLES AND MUSHROOMS AT-A-GLANCE

VARIETY	NUTRIENTS	GOOD FOR
Garlic	Vitamin C, calcium, potassium, manganese, selenium, zinc.	Immunity – natural antibacterial, antiseptic, antiviral, decongestant, lowering LDL cholesterol.
Leeks	Vitamins B6, C, manganese, iron.	Cleansing, diuretic, antispasmodic, helping to heal stomach ulcers.
Red beetroot (beets)	Folic acid, Vitamin C, beta-carotene, manganese, potassium.	Stimulating liver detoxification, intestinal cleanser, preventing constipation, lowering cholesterol levels, antioxidant.
Red onions	Vitamins B6, C, manganese, iron.	Natural antibiotic, antiviral, easing asthma and allergies, controlling blood sugar levels, nervous system.
Shallots	Vitamins B2, B3, B6, C, iron.	Energy production, cardiovascular system.
Spring onions (scallions)	Vitamins B2, B3, B6, C, iron, manganese, potassium.	Natural antiseptic, antispasmodic, calming to the digestion.
Wild garlic	Vitamin B6, magnesium, manganese, selenium, sulphur, zinc.	Antimicrobial, antiseptic, lowering blood pressure and cholesterol, bone health, heart health.
White onions	Vitamins B6, C, manganese.	Antiseptic, antibiotic, natural antihistamine, blood sugar control.
Yellow beetroot (beets)	Folic acid, vitamin C, manganese, potassium.	Stimulating liver detoxification, intestinal cleanser, preventing constipation, lowering cholesterol levels, antioxidant.
Mushrooms	Vitamins B2, B3, B5, copper, selenium, potassium.	Low-GI, sustained release energy, immunity.

AVOID white, black and sweet potatoes, parsnips, yams and Jerusalem artichokes.

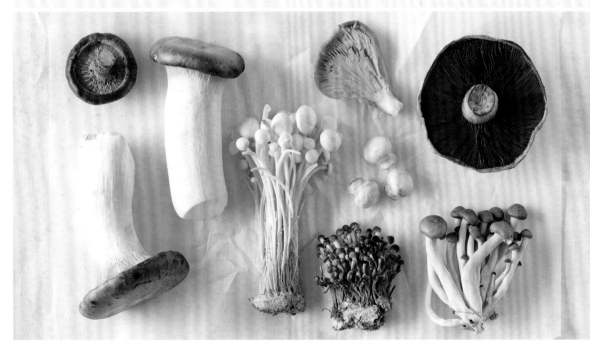

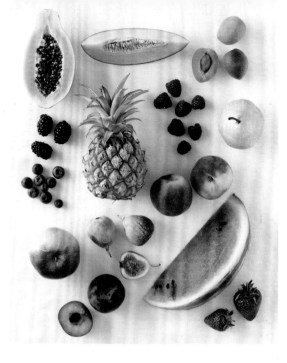

Always blanch salad vegetables to break down and soften their cellulose and release their nutrients – don't eat them raw. For more information on how to blanch vegetables turn to the salads chapter (see pages 196–199). Salad leaves can remain raw after washing and draining; firm vegetables, such as broccoli and asparagus, should be lightly steamed, baked or roasted.

As no grains are permitted on the Plan, eat more vegetables with some protein at every meal to manage your blood sugar levels and stop you feeling hungry.

EAT YOUR GREENS

Whilst a rainbow of coloured vegetables is included on this Plan, the concentration of green vegetables constitutes the greatest proportion of the total collection. These are the most nutrient-dense ones, which contain an array of antioxidant vitamins and minerals to protect all the organs in the body, and provide all the nutrients needed for energy production at a cellular level. Most are packed with vitamin C (see the chart on page 25), which we have to get on a daily basis from the food we eat as it cannot be stored in the body. It is considered one of the most essential protective vitamins, working with the other antioxidants to help repair and regenerate the lining of the gut as well as neutralizing potential toxins.

Fruits

The fruits that are allowed on the Plan are all easy to break down and cause the least fermentation in the gut. Most of these are included in breakfast dishes – eating fruit on an empty stomach reduces the likelihood of bloating and wind. Some of the salads also include fruits, and it's better to eat these at lunchtime rather than later in the day to avoid bloating and discomfort.

Ripe fruits, including apples, pears, peaches and berries, are preferable to unripe ones as you can digest these more easily (see the list of permitted fruits overleaf on page 28). All fruits are rich in protective antioxidants, which help ward off toxins, potential pathogenic bacteria and viruses (see pages 14–15).

All the vitamin A in fruits is found in the form of beta-carotene, which is not only one of the most potent carotenoids but also great for your skin. In the same way that these antioxidants are present in the fruits to protect them from environmental toxins, they also protect the internal 'skin' of the digestive tract (the epithelial lining).

The B vitamins in fruit are all involved in energy production at a cellular level and are responsible for all the functions in the brain, adrenal gland (manages stress) and thyroid (stimulates metabolism).

Carbs to curb

The list of carbs to avoid eating on the Plan includes:

Sugars and sweeteners: agar-agar, agave syrup, arrowroot, aspartame, balsamic vinegar, corn syrup, golden syrup, carob, chocolates, cocoa powder, molasses, pectin (in apples), fructose powder.

Grains: amaranth, barley, buckwheat, bulgar, cereals, couscous, all grain flours, millet, oats, pasta, quinoa, rye, semolina, tapioca, wheat and wheat-germ.

Fruits: dates, raisins, grapes, all dried fruit, canned fruits, apple juice and fruit juices of all kinds.

Vegetables: broad beans, sweetcorn, Jerusalem artichokes, okra, parsnips, potatoes (all), soya beans, preserved or canned vegetables, turnips and yams.

Legumes: baked beans, black-eyed beans, cannellini beans, chickpeas and kidney beans.

FRUITS AT-A-GLANCE

VARIETY	NUTRIENTS	GOOD FOR
Apples	Vitamin C, bioflavonoids, calcium, magnesium.	Helping with absorption of iron, relieving constipation, beneficial gut bacteria, removing toxins.
Apricots	Beta-carotene, carotenoids, vitamin C, potassium.	Promoting healthy bowels, iron absorption.
Avocados	Vitamins B6, E, K, folic acid,	Improving skin tone and moisture, lowering LDL cholesterol levels.
Blackberries	Vitamins C, K, bioflavonoids, copper, manganese.	Cleansing blood, relieving diarrhoea, boosting immunity.
Blueberries	Vitamins C, E, beta-carotene.	Antioxidants, reducing risk of heart disease and age-related degenerative diseases, boosting immunity, eye health.
Cherries	Vitamins C, K, bioflavonoids, potassium.	Anti-inflammatory, easing headaches, treating gout and arthritis, regulating sleep patterns.
Cranberries	Vitamin C, bioflavonoids, manganese.	Antibacterial, antioxidant, supporting digestive and urinary tract and cardiovascular and immune systems.
Elderberries	Beta-carotene, flavone, vitamins A, K and C.	Lowering cholesterol, boosting immune system, heart health, antibacterial and fighting viral infections.
Figs	Beta-carotene, vitamin C, calcium.	Natural laxative for sluggish bowels, clearing toxins.
Nectarines	Beta-carotene, vitamins A, C, beta-carotene, potassium.	Aiding digestion, regulating pH, boosting immunity, skin health.
Olives	Beta-carotene, vitamin E, calcium, iron.	Liver and gall bladder support, skin health.
Pears	Vitamins C, K, beta-carotene, copper.	Diuretic, thyroid function, removing toxins from digestive tract, fibre.
Plums	Vitamins C, K, beta-carotene, bioflavonoids.	Boosting immunity, increasing absorption of iron.
Pomegranates	Vitamins B5, C, bioflavonoids, potassium.	Antioxidant, lowering blood pressure, improving blood circulation and heart health, antibacterial, boosting immunity.
Raspberries	Vitamins B2, C, folic acid, magnesium, manganese.	Immunity, antioxidants, brain and cognitive function.
Rhubarb	Vitamins C, K, carotenoids, calcium, potassium.	Improving blood circulation, digestion and cardiovascular health.
Strawberries	Vitamin C, bioflavonoids, manganese, potassium.	Boosting energy, relieving eczema and asthma, anti-ageing antioxidants.
Tomatoes	Vitamins C, K, beta-carotene, folic acid, lycopene, calcium.	Antiseptic, alkaline, reducing liver inflammation, protecting against prostate, lung and stomach cancers.
Watermelon	Vitamins B1, B6, C, beta-carotene, magnesium, potassium.	Cardiovascular health, natural diuretic, alkaline.
White currants	Vitamins C, E, potassium, fibre.	Fibre, antispasmodic, antioxidant, immunity and skin health.
White peaches	Vitamin C, beta-carotene, carotenoids, bioflavonoids, copper.	Alkaline, cleansing for kidneys and bladder.

AVOID all canned and juiced fruits and any dried fruit with added sulphur or which has not been soaked overnight.

Fats

Not all fats are considered equal, so it is vital that you understand how they perform in the body – no less than 60 per cent of the brain is comprised of fats, and all the nerves and the entire neurological system depend on the right intake of essential fats to function optimally. The benefits of consuming good fats on the Plan include improved mood, concentration and focus, lustrous hair and soft, supple skin, as well as boosting the body's immunity through the fat-soluble nutrients they carry: vitamins A, D, E and K. Most of the fats that are found in foods are a combination of essential fats (monounsaturated and polyunsaturated) and saturated fats, so it is not simply a question of cutting out one and replacing it with another.

SATURATED FATS

On the Plan, you should always consume fats in their natural state – i.e. by leaving the visible fat on meat and poultry (the skin), tossing salads with dressings that are made with essential fats (e.g. walnut oil), and consuming oily fish, such as salmon and mackerel. Many of the protein foods we eat contain fat, some of which are saturated fats. These are found mainly in animal protein sources as well as coconut and palm oil. Saturated fats used to be considered unhealthy, as it was thought that they could increase the level of 'bad' LDL (low-density lipoprotein) cholesterol in the blood and arteries, which possibly contributes to heart disease and stroke. However, we now know that it is the combination of saturated fats and sugar that causes arterial plaque, leading to these degenerative diseases, and not the fat by itself. Without the sugars, saturated fats are healthy, leading to feeling less hungry and weight loss.

Found in red meat, poultry, coconut oil, palm oil, butter and ghee (clarified butter), saturated fat is rich in CLA, (conjugated linoleic acid – see the panel on the right), which helps to break down stored fat in the body. It is the combination of good-quality proteins (from grass-fed livestock, for example) together with vegetables and salad ingredients that help the healing and repair of the body and, in particular, the digestive tract.

THE ESSENTIAL FATS

The two main groups of essential fatty acids – Omega-3 and Omega-6 – are known as essential because the body can't make them itself, so we have to get them from the foods that we eat. Both groups complement each other in their benefits (although the Omega-6 fats can promote inflammation), yet both are required to balance each other out. They are essential for brain health, the heart and cardiovascular systems, and for literally 'oiling' our joints – people on a very low-fat, no-fat diet are more prone to rheumatoid arthritis or other inflammatory joint conditions, eczema or psoriasis, which are also conditions of inflammation.

Omega-3 in its richest source is found primarily in oily cold-water fish (fish that swim in deep waters like mackerel, sardines and salmon). It is also present in white fish, including sea bass, bream, haddock, pollock, cod and halibut, as well as in seaweed and algae. Additionally, it is present in the fat of pasture-fed meat and in organic eggs (hence the recommendation to always choose organic) as well as CLA (see below).

The importance of CLA

In the last 10 years or so, it has been determined that the highest level of CLA (conjugated linoleic acid) is to be found in red meat. CLA is one of the essential fatty acids of the anti-inflammatory Omega-3 group, and it helps 'burn' stored fat. It is also called the 'skinny' fat, as burning fat is one of its main functions. Ironically, a good-quality meat burger will never make anyone fat – it's only the sweetened bun and all the condiments that pile on the pounds! Whilst several weight-loss supplements now include CLA, nothing is as effective as getting it from the food you eat.

Saturated fats are the best ones to use for cooking, as they are robust and don't damage easily, so you can use goose fat, dripping (from cows) and lard (from pigs), butter and ghee (clarified butter) as these won't turn into trans fats (rancid, damaging fats) when heated. For a vegetarian option, choose coconut oil instead. It really is the best oil for cooking but use culinary-quality oil to avoid everything tasting of coconut!

FATS AT-A-GLANCE

FAT	NUTRIENTS	GOOD FOR
ANIMAL-BASED		
Butter, ghee	Saturated fat, vitamins A, D, E and K, B12, chromium, zinc.	Immunity, antioxidants, balancing blood sugar levels and reducing cravings.
Duck, goose	Monounsaturated fat, Omega-6, vitamin E, palmitoleic acid.	Stable cooking oil, fighting intestinal microbials, anti-bacterial.
Lard and dripping (pig)	Monounsaturated fat, Omega-6, vitamin E, palmitoleic acid.	Stable cooking oil at high temperature, antimicrobial, weight loss.
Beef and lamb	50% saturated fat, 40% monounsaturated fat (Omega-3 and -6, CLA), palmitoleic acid.	Weight loss, heart health, antimicrobial.
Fish: All white fish, salmon, sardines, anchovies	Omega-3, DHA, vitamin E, calcium	Immunity, brain health, concentration, memory, nervous system.
Shellfish: Crab, lobster, mussels, clams, shrimp	Zinc, selenium, calcium	Immunity, bone health, thyroid (metabolism), memory.
PLANT-BASED		
Coconut	Monounsaturated, lauric acid (also found in human breast milk), vitamin E.	Cooking, antimicrobial/antifungal, hair, skin and nails – no rancidity at room temperature.
Chia	Highest plant-source Omega-3, vitamin E, fibre, protein, vitamins B1, B2, B3, manganese, magnesium, zinc.	Complete food, anti-inflammatory, brain, focus, concentration, hair and skin health.
Avocado	Vitamins B6, C, E, K, Omega-3, monounsaturated and oleic fats.	Antioxidants, heart health, immunity, hair, skin – use cold-pressed oil only.
Olive	Vitamins C, E, Omega-3, oleic fat.	Antioxidant, hair, skin, heart, cardiovascular – use cold-pressed oil and cook at low temperatures.
Pumpkin seeds	Omega-3 and -6 polyunsaturated and monounsaturated essential fats, vitamin E.	Antioxidant, immunity, prostate health.
Sunflower seeds	Low-saturated fat/high oleic fat, Omega-3 and -6 essential fats, vitamins B1, B2, B6.	Weight-loss, lowering LDL cholesterol, anti-anxiety – use cold-pressed oil in dressings only.
Sesame	Selenium, Omega-3 and -6 essntial fats, vitamin E, low-saturated.	Skin and hair, immunity, anti-oxidant, heart health.
Walnut	Vitamin E, copper, manganese, Omega-3 essential fat, magnesium.	Heart health, skin, hair, brain – mood and concentration.

AVOID 'false' fats, including margarine and vegetable oil/spreadable butters.

Whilst these fats can also be found in nuts and seeds, this source of Omega-3 is less easy for your body to absorb and use than animal-derived fats, which is why animal-sourced foods account for so many of the recipes in this book. The main uses of Omega-3 are related to heart and brain health. With potent anti-inflammatory properties, it is essential for preventing atherosclerosis – plaque formation from excess LDL cholesterol and calcium deposits, which causes stroke and heart disease. Omega-3 also helps create serotonin (the 'happy-factor' neurotransmitter which is synthesized in the gut and utilized by the brain), supporting such functions as good mood, concentration and focus, satisfaction, pleasure and laughter.

The Omega-6 group, which is found in nuts, seeds and their oils, is required for brain and muscle development, cellular growth throughout the body, healing and repair, and it complements the Omega-3 fats. Both groups work in tandem, although in reality the ratio of Omega-6:Omega-3 tends to be 20:1 when it should be 2:1!

Coconut

Coconut is being heralded as the best vegetarian fat of all for the following reasons:

- It helps to balance blood sugar levels by slowing down the release of glucose into the bloodstream.
- It reduces cravings (for sweet foods).
- It supports immunity as a potent antibacterial/antifungal treatment in its oil, flesh, water and milk.
- It supports thyroid function, elevating metabolic rate, and producing more energy.
- It helps to reduce blood pressure and supports heart health.
- It improves the suppleness of the skin, and increases hair volume and shine.

This is most likely due to people's over-consumption of pre-packed and processed meats and snacks, and is a major reason for eating fresh foods in preference to processed ones.

There is a third group of essential fats that is known as mono- (single) unsaturated fats; these are semi-solid when they are chilled. They also contribute to heart health as well as reducing atherosclerotic plaque by stimulating the release of bile. Olive oil, groundnut, avocado and macadamia nut oils fall within this category. Rich in flavour, these oils should be used in a cold-pressed state for salad dressings only.

ALMOND MILK

You can make nutritious non-dairy 'milks' from nuts. To make almond milk, simply soak 150g (5oz/1 cup) raw unsalted almonds in a bowl of water overnight. They will plump up as they absorb the water. The following day, drain the almonds and rinse thoroughly under cold running water. Place the almonds and 500ml (16fl oz/2 cups) filtered water in a blender and blitz at high speed for 2 minutes. Line a strainer with some cheesecloth and place it over a measuring jug. Press the almond mixture through the strainer – you should end up with about 500ml (16fl oz/2 cups). Store in a sealed container in the fridge for up to 2 days.

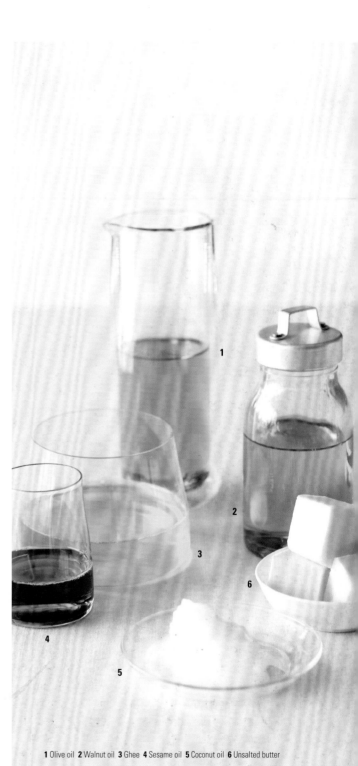

1 Olive oil **2** Walnut oil **3** Ghee **4** Sesame oil **5** Coconut oil **6** Unsalted butter

Herbs and spices

As well as having specific roles in the culinary field, every herb and spice also possesses extremely potent nutritional benefits. Some are more flavoursome than others, so take care when using them for the first time to decide which ones appeal to you the most, as your nutritional needs also dictate the herbs and spices you will want to eat. There is information below and overleaf on the nutritional benefits of all the herbs and spices used in the recipes in this book.

Many herbs and spices are available dried as well as fresh. The dried varieties tend to be more intensely flavoured and therefore they are often used in smaller quantities for flavouring dishes. You can grow fresh ones yourself in pots on the patio or your kitchen windowsill.

Herbs

Basil Potent and refreshing in taste, this Mediterranean herb is packed with antioxidants that protect at a cellular level. Basil also has antibacterial and anti-inflammatory properties and contains the heart-healthy nutrients beta-carotene and magnesium. Use it in soups, smoothies, salads, tomato dishes and pesto.

Bay leaf One of the oldest and best-recognized spices, the bay leaf is rich in beta-carotene, vitamin C, zinc and selenium – primary antioxidants. It is antiseptic and protects the internal and external skin. Eaten regularly, it can also protect you against insect bites. Use it in soups, casseroles, fish, meat and vegetable dishes.

Chives Fresh and tart in flavour, chives are part of the allium family (onions, garlic, leeks) and are known for their antibacterial/fungal/viral properties, and cleansing the gastrointestinal (GI) tract. They also help to reduce cholesterol production when it's too high. They have more vitamins A and K than any other allium plant. Use them liberally in soups, salads and with fish.

Coriander (cilantro) leaves and stalks Found in many Mediterranean and Asian dishes, coriander (cilantro) contains one of the highest levels of vitamin K, which is important for healthy bones, as well as vitamins C and A for eye health and repairing the gut. This herb is known

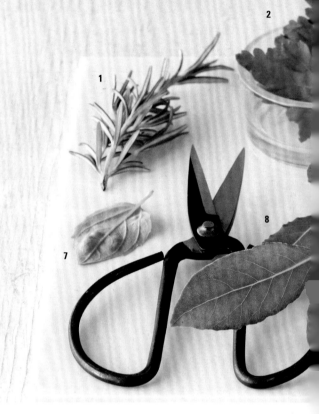

1 Rosemary 2 Flat-leaf parsley 3 Tarragon 4 Thyme 5 Sage
6 Chives 7 Basil 8 Bay leaf 9 Dill 10 Chervil 11 Coriander (cilantro)
12 Mint 13 Rosemary flowers

to have antibacterial properties. People love or hate its distinctive flavour. It is good in soups, juices, fish dishes, vegetables and many Asian and Mexican dishes.

Mint This herb has a fresh, cleansing flavour and possesses gut-soothing, antibacterial and antimicrobial properties, helping ease indigestion, stomach pain and bloating. Drink it as a tea, infuse in drinking water, or use with lamb, fish, soups and salads.

Parsley This is known as the best natural toothpaste of all – for its cleansing effects against bacteria in the mouth. Parsley is also packed with vitamin C, folic acid and flavonoids – all recognized as potent antioxidants that support heart health.

Rosemary A pungent aromatic herb that stimulates the

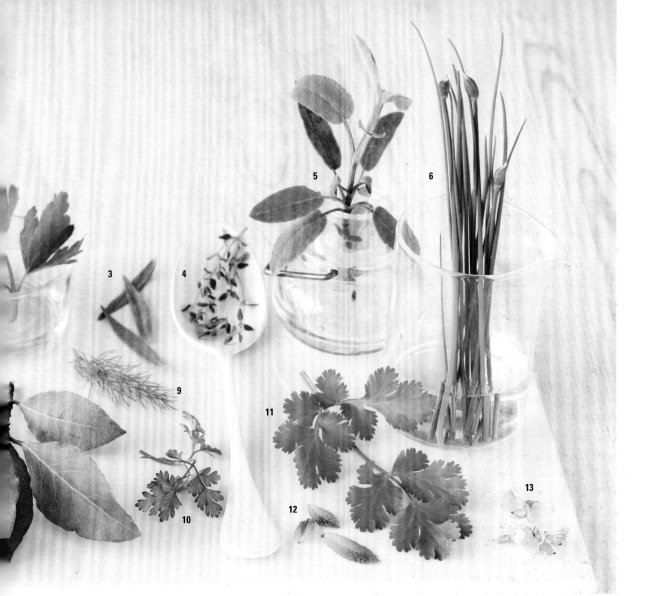

nervous system, creating alertness and concentration; too much, however, may cause anxiety. It increases blood flow to the heart, head and brain, and its anti-inflammatory properties help people with asthma and breathing difficulties. Use with fish as well as meats, and as a flavouring for water and dressings.

Rosemary flowers As well as being delicately flavoured, the flowers provide an intense array of antiseptic, anti-allergic and anti-fungal compounds that warrant their inclusion in your salads, or you can use them in herbal teas and as a garnish for topping soups.

Sage Part of the rosemary family, the rosmarinic acid in sage is easily absorbed by the gastrointestinal (GI) tract, creating anti-inflammatory responses in the bloodstream. It has stimulating effects on neurons in the brain, aiding concentration and memory. Use liberally in soups and casseroles and with chicken.

Tarragon This herb increases bile production, which makes fats more digestible, and provides potent antioxidants to support the GI function and eyesight. Its light and lemony flavour (especially Turkish tarragon) is cleansing to the palate, and it helps balance female hormones and is beneficial for heart health.

Thyme Delicate in flavour and potent in antioxidants, this herb has abundant antimicrobial properties and helps to boost levels of DHA (a vital essential fatty acid) in the brain. Use it in poultry and fish dishes, casseroles, soups and herbal teas.

Spices

Cardamom Excellent for easing indigestion and digestive problems. It helps combat infections by eliminating waste and toxins through the kidneys.

Cinnamon Regulates blood sugar levels by enhancing the effect of insulin. It has potent anti-inflammatory properties and is good for joint pain, irritable bowel syndrome and skin problems.

Chilli powder This can aid weight loss by boosting your metabolism and releasing endorphins to enhance your mood. Great for heart health – thinning blood and improving cholesterol levels. Anti-fungal and antibacterial, chillies are packed with antioxidants and are proven to lower blood sugar levels.

Cloves Packed with antioxidants, vitamin A and beta-carotene, Omega-3 fatty acids and vitamins, cloves are anti-inflammatory, antiseptic and anti-flatulent. They help relieve indigestion and constipation and contain potassium for controlling blood pressure.

Coriander seeds Aromatic, sweet and citrusy, these are rich in antioxidants and vitamins A and C, as well as cell-protective oils when crushed.

Fennel seeds With their sweet anise flavour, fennel seeds can reduce menstrual cramps and help regulate hormones. They contain numerous flavonoid antioxidants, which remove harmful free radicals from the body, protecting it from cancers, infection, ageing and degenerative neurological diseases.

Fenugreek This staple Indian spice has antiviral properties, relieving colds and flu. It helps reduce irritability during menopause and PMS. It can be used as a laxative, digestive, and as a remedy for coughs and bronchitis. Fenugreek seeds are high in soluble fibre, which helps to lower blood sugar, making them key in improving the symptoms that are associated with both Type 1 and Type 2 diabetes.

Ginger A warm, aromatic spice which is known for its ability to soothe the respiratory tract and treat common colds and coughs. Gingerols, the potent anti-inflammatory compounds found in ginger, help to reduce arthritic, joint and muscle pain while preventing gas formation and aiding digestion. Ginger is believed to relieve nausea and vomiting during pregnancy.

Juniper Like other bitter spices, juniper has the ability to improve your digestion as bitters cause saliva, digestive enzymes and stomach acid secretions to increase. It also has diuretic properties and is known to relieve symptoms of bloating and water retention as well as being high in antioxidants.

Mustard seeds (white) These are an excellent source of selenium and magnesium, with anti-inflammatory properties, helping to control asthma and cold symptoms and relieving arthritic and muscle pain. Contain immune-boosting minerals iron and copper, which increase the body's ability to fight disease.

Nutmeg A mood-boosting sweet, aromatic spice containing potassium, calcium, iron, magnesium and zinc. Also rich in B-complex vitamins, vitamin C, folic acid and beta-carotene. It stimulates the brain, improves concentration, helps eliminate stress, fatigue, anxiety and depression and can be used to relieve painful aching joints and muscles. It also relieves digestive problems and improves sleep.

Peppercorns (black) These stimulate hydrochloric acid secretion in the stomach, improving digestion and preventing the formation of intestinal gas, diarrhoea and constipation. They can also promote sweating and urination, removing toxins from the body.

Poppy seeds (black) The oil seeds derived from the poppy plant contain calcium, copper, phosphorus and manganese – all minerals that strengthen and protect your bones but also help your heart and nervous system function. Mild in flavour and rich in dietary fibre, poppy seeds can also lower cholesterol levels.

Turmeric Known for its healing properties, turmeric is used to treat wounds and skin conditions such as psoriasis. It also provides potent antibacterial, antiviral and antifungal properties as well as anti-ageing effects as it neutralizes free radicals, which can lead to wrinkles. It improves liver detoxification and also supports the immune, digestive and nervous system.

Vanilla This spice has calming properties that can help reduce anxiety. A great source of antioxidants, it is also anti-inflammatory and antibacterial, helping to heal wounds and soothe skin infections. Vanilla is packed with B-vitamins, which are key to maintaining healthy-looking skin.

1 Whole nutmeg
2 Whole cloves
3 Ground turmeric
4 Caraway seeds
5 Poppy seeds
6 Fennel seeds
7 Ground cinnamon
8 Green cardamom pods
9 Juniper berries
10 Coriander seeds
11 Paprika
12 Vanilla pod
13 Cumin seeds
14 Star anise
15 Chilli powder
16 Cinnamon stick
17 Ground ginger
18 Allspice
19 Pink peppercorns
20 Black peppercorns

Finishing salts

Good-quality salt will help you to absorb the nutrients in the foods you eat. Complex salt, such as pink Himalayan salt, provides many minerals aside from sodium. These recipes show how you can use flavoured salts as an enhancing condiment.

Lime zest, kaffir lime & lemongrass salt

Makes: 140g (4½oz)

15g (½oz) lime zest, finely grated

10g (½oz) fresh kaffir lime leaf

15g (½oz) lemongrass stalk, peeled

100g (3½oz) Maldon sea salt flakes

40g (1½oz/3 tbsp) pink Himalayan salt

Prepare the lime zest:

Option 1: Preheat the oven to 110°C, Gas mark ¼ (non fan). Line a baking tray with parchment paper and sprinkle the lime zest over it. Cook in the preheated oven for 3 hours.

Option 2 (quick and easy method): lay a piece of parchment paper over a microwave dish and sprinkle with the lime zest. Make 5 blasts of 20 seconds at full power, mixing the zest between blasts to avoid any lumps.

Chop the kaffir lime leaf until finely shredded. Finely chop the lemongrass. Mix them with the lime zest and salt. Store in an airtight container in a cool place for up to 3 months.

Tangerine, cumin, fennel & chipotle salt

Makes: 150g (5oz)

30g (1oz) tangerine zest, finely grated

1 tsp cumin seeds, toasted

1 tsp fennel seeds, toasted

1 tbsp dried chipotle chilli, finely chopped

100g (3½oz/scant ½ cup) Maldon sea salt flakes

40g (1½oz/3 tbsp) pink Himalayan salt

Prepare the tangerine zest:

Option 1: Preheat the oven to 110°C, Gas mark ¼ (non fan). Line a baking tray with parchment paper and sprinkle the tangerine zest over it. Cook in the preheated oven for 3 hours.

Option 2 (quick and easy method): lay a piece of parchment paper over a microwave dish and sprinkle with the tangerine zest. Make 5 blasts of 20 seconds at full power, mixing the zest between blasts to avoid lumps.

Mix the toasted cumin and fennel seeds together and crumble them in a spice grinder. Mix the tangerine zest, pulverized seeds, chipotle chilli and salt together. Store in an airtight container in a cool place for up to 3 months.

Orange, juniper, rosemary & thyme salt

Makes: 175g (6oz)

50g (2oz) orange zest, finely grated

12–15 juniper berries

½ bunch of fresh lemon thyme sprigs

¼ bunch of fresh rosemary sprigs

100g (3½oz/scant ½ cup) Maldon sea salt flakes

Prepare the orange zest:

Option 1: Preheat the oven to 110°C, Gas mark ¼ (non fan). Line a baking tray with parchment paper and sprinkle the orange zest over it. Cook in the preheated oven for 3 hours.

Option 2 (quick and easy method): lay a piece of parchment paper over a microwave dish and sprinkle with the orange zest. Make 5 blasts of 20 seconds at full power, mixing the zest between blasts to avoid any lumps.

Crush the juniper berries in a spice grinder. Pick the leaves and flowers, if possible, off the lemon thyme. Pick the leaves off the rosemary and chop as small as possible.

Mix into the salt. Store in an airtight container in a cool place for up to three months.

Five-spice & grapefruit salt

Makes: 150g (5oz)

30g (1oz) grapefruit zest, finely grated

100g (3½oz/scant ½ cup) Maldon sea salt flakes

1 star anise

2 cloves

1cm (½in) cinnamon stick

½ tsp Szechuan peppercorns

1 tsp fennel seeds, toasted and ground to powder

Prepare the grapefruit zest:

Option 1: Preheat the oven to 110°C, Gas mark ¼ (non fan). Line a baking tray with parchment paper and sprinkle the grapefruit zest over it. Cook in the preheated oven for 3 hours.

Option 2 (quick and easy method): lay a piece of parchment paper over a microwave dish and sprinkle with the grapefruit zest. Make 5 blasts of 20 seconds at full power, mixing the zest between blasts to avoid lumps.

Mix the grapefruit zest with the other ingredients. Store in an airtight container in a cool place for up to 3 months.

Lemon, paprika & garlic salt

Prepare the lemon zest:

Option 1: Preheat the oven to 110°C, Gas mark ¼ (non fan). Line a baking tray with some parchment paper and sprinkle the lemon zest over it. Cook in the preheated oven for 3 hours.

Option 2 (quick and easy method): lay a piece of parchment paper over a microwave dish and sprinkle with the lemon zest. Make 5 blasts of 20 seconds at full power, mixing the zest between blasts to avoid lumps.

Mix the lemon zest with all the other ingredients. Store in an airtight container in a cool place for up to 3 months.

Makes: 150g (5oz)

20g (¾oz) lemon zest, finely grated

3 garlic cloves, sliced

1 tsp smoked hot paprika

100g (3½oz/scant ½ cup) Maldon sea salt flakes

Orange, juniper, rosemary & thyme salt

Five-spice & grapefruit salt

Tangerine, cumin, fennel & chipotle salt

Lime zest, kaffir lime & lemongrass salt

Fermented foods

We recommend having some fermented foods prior to eating every meal. Germans, Poles and Russians have been doing this for years, eating pickled and fermented foods for their digestive benefits, as have the Japanese in the form of picked cucumbers, onions and radish. In fact, in Korea, Kimchi, or pickled cabbage, is the national dish. Fermented foods provide health benefits through the way in which their inherent bacteria, yeasts and moulds all 'predigest' foods, breaking down the carbohydrates, fats and proteins that are ingested in the ensuing meal to create probiotics that introduce beneficial bacteria into the digestive system.

WHY YOU SHOULD EAT FERMENTED FOODS

Fermented foods are an acquired taste for some people, but most of us get used to them within a couple of days. Slightly acidic to the taste-buds, pickled vegetables are, in fact, alkaline once they have been digested. However, it is their role in stimulating the hydrochloric acid in the stomach that is so important. As discussed earlier, stress interferes with the stomach's production of hydrochloric acid (with the release of cortisol from the adrenal glands), which shuts down all but what is essential for the 'fight or flight' mechanism. In a highly stressed situation, the digestion is put on hold in favour of more important bodily functions. When the digestive system isn't working well from the top end, it adversely affects what goes on in the small and large intestines, too.

SMART SAUERKRAUTS

Traditional sauerkraut, as made in Germany and Poland, uses cabbage as its base. This is because the isothiocynate (sulphur containing) compounds in cabbage contain cancer-fighting compounds. This is the most common of all sauerkrauts and it can be sourced in ready-made versions in supermarkets. However, whilst better than none at all, these are nowhere as tasty or effective as home-made versions, as you will discover once you have tried both of them. With his passion for delicious, healthy food, Adam has produced several alternative recipes after researching dishes from different countries around the world, and it is worth trying the different types to see which you prefer. We have named these recipes 'smart sauerkrauts' as they 'switch on' the body's digestive system by stimulating the stomach to produce acids in the presence of vitamin B12.

Pickled sauerkrauts are made by cutting and crushing raw vegetables to release the fluids they contain, then layering them with salt (and other flavourings) to create a fermentation that breaks the vegetables down into a product that is more easily digestible. We favour monosaccharides (the most basic units of carbohydrates) on this Plan, so it is important that you eat some at the start of every meal. The following recipes can be made two to three weeks before being consumed but the longer they ferment, the more their cellulose breaks down, creating a stronger flavour. They are fermented at room temperature until cooked (see page 41) and then put into the fridge, where they stop fermenting. Their pungent odour comes from the lactic acid that is produced by the fermentation. This also creates an abundance of 'friendly' or beneficial bacteria – such an important part of the Plan for increasing digestive health, stimulating the immunity in the gut, and reducing the incidence of IBS (irritable bowel syndrome).

BITTERS AND APPLE CIDER VINEGAR

Using bitter tinctures to help break down food in the stomach is vital. Take them in a little water before every main meal. Bitters are available from all good health food stores, but apple cider vinegar is the old-fashioned but still effective alternative. A scant half teaspoon stirred into a small mug of warm water is ample.

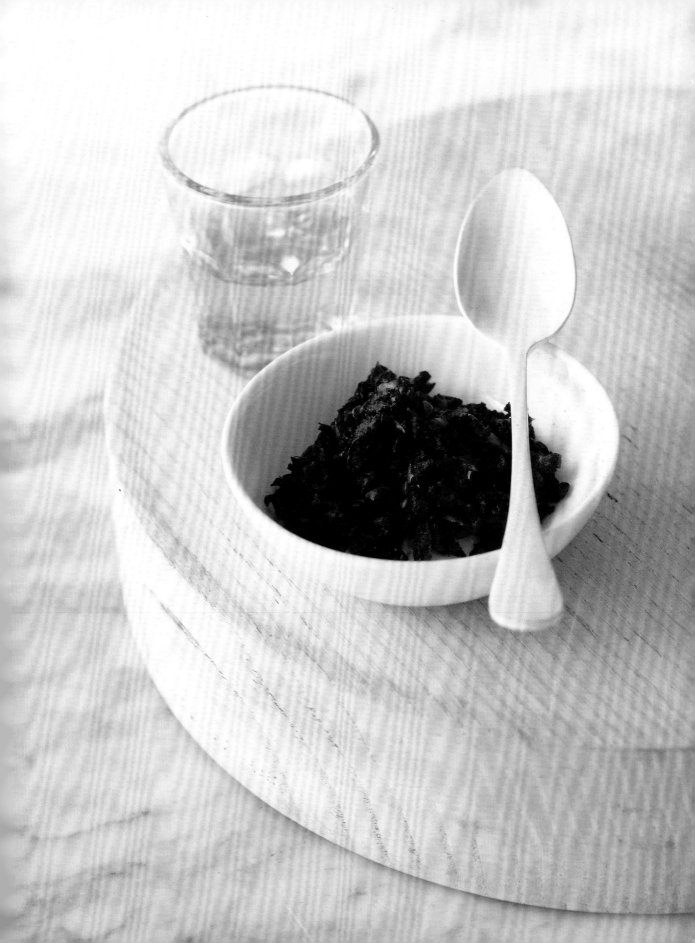

CLOCKWISE FROM BACK LEFT: Thai fermented napa; Bok chi; Borski kraut (and in bowl, foreground); Fermented fennel, savoy cabbage & pimento; Sproutchi kraut; Fermented red cabbage, apple, juniper & coriander

Make your own smart sauerkrauts

Whilst you can buy commercial sauerkraut, it is best to make your own. These recipes need upwards of three weeks to ferment, which is not always practical, but well worth it in the early stages of the Plan.

Bok chi

Makes: 2 litres (3½ pints/8 cups)

200g (7oz) red (bell) pepper, deseeded and roughly chopped

30g (1oz) fresh red chilli

50g (2oz) fresh root ginger, peeled and chopped

15g (½oz) garlic cloves, peeled and chopped

15g (½oz/1 tbsp) good-quality sea salt

20ml (4 tsp) Thai fish sauce (nam pla)

700g (1½lb) pak choi, sliced 1cm (½in) wide

2kg (4lb 7oz) mouli, peeled and cut into 1cm (½in) dice

100g (3½oz) spring onions (scallions), shredded

Sterilize a 2-litre (3½-pint) Kilner jar: wash the jar in soapy water and dry it. Pour boiling water into the jar, empty it and place on a baking tray in a preheated cool oven at 140°C, 275F, Gas mark 1, until it's completely dry.

Blend the red (bell) pepper, chilli, ginger, garlic, sea salt and Thai fish sauce in a food processor until smooth.

In a separate large mixing bowl add the pak choi, mouli and spring onions. Pour the red pepper mixture over the top, using a rolling pin to smash the pak choi and other ingredients, so they release some of their natural juice. The salt will help as it naturally draws moisture out of the food.

When the mixture in the bowl is covered with a small amount of liquid it is ready to be spooned into the sterilized jar. Fill the jar, leaving a 3cm (1in) gap at the top. Using a plastic spatula, clean around the top of the jar, ensuring the mixture is submerged under the liquid. Close the lid and leave at room temperature out of direct sunlight for 3 weeks before checking for fermentation (see page 41). When checking (after 3 weeks), use a clean spoon and taste to see if the vegetables have started to ferment.

Store in the refrigerator with the lid on. The fermentation will slow down at cooler temperatures and will last for up to 1 month.

Sproutchi kraut

Makes: 2 litres (3½ pints/8 cups)

2kg (4lb 3½oz) Brussels sprouts

175g (6oz) shallots, finely sliced

40g (1½oz/3 tbsp) sea salt

20g (¾oz) whole yellow mustard seeds

25g (1oz) thyme, leaves stripped from the stalks

Shred the sprouts in a food processor. Put them in a large mixing bowl with all the other ingredients. Using a rolling pin, smash the sprouts and the other ingredients to release some of their natural juices. The salt also helps to naturally draw out the moisture of the food.

When the mixture in the bowl is covered with a small amount of liquid it is ready to be spooned into a sterilized 2-litre (3½-pint) jar (see recipe above).

Fill the jar but leave a 3cm (1in) gap at the top. Using a plastic spatula, clean around the top of the jar to make sure the mixture is submerged under the liquid. Close the jar and leave at room temperature out of direct sunlight for 3 weeks before checking for fermentation (see above).

When checking the sproutchi kraut, use a clean spoon to taste whether the vegetables have started to ferment.

After opening, store in the refrigerator with the lid on. The fermentation will slow down at cooler temperatures and the mixture will last for up to 1 month.

Fermented fennel, savoy cabbage & pimento

Makes: 2 litres (3½ pints/8 cups)

900g (2lb) fennel bulb, finely shredded

1.25kg (2lb 12oz) Savoy cabbage, finely shredded

10g (½oz) whole pimento, ground with a pestle and mortar

30g (1¼oz/2 tbsp) sea salt

Sterilize a 2-litre (3½-pint) Kilner jar (see page 41).

Put all the ingredients in a large mixing bowl. Using a rolling pin, smash the fennel and other ingredients so that they release some of their natural juices. The salt helps as it naturally draws out the moisture of food.

When the mixture has a small amount of liquid covering it in the bowl, it is ready to be spooned into the sterilized jar. Fill the jar but leave a 3cm (1in) gap at the top. Using a plastic spatula, clean around the top of the jar, ensuring that the mixture is submerged under the liquid. Close the lid and leave at room temperature for 3 weeks before checking for fermentation. When checking, use a clean spoon and taste if the vegetables have started to ferment.

Store in the refrigerator with the lid on. Fermentation will slow down at cooler temperatures and will last a good few weeks.

Fermented red cabbage, apple, juniper & coriander

Makes: 2 litres (3½ pints/8 cups)

3kg (6lb 10oz) red cabbage, shredded

20 juniper berries, ground with a pestle and mortar

30 coriander seeds, ground with a pestle and mortar

300g (10oz) Granny Smith apples, cored and grated

60g (2½oz/¼ cup) sea salt

Sterilize a 2-litre (3½-pint) Kilner jar (see page 41).

Put all the ingredients in a large mixing bowl. Using a rolling pin, smash the fennel and cabbage so they release some of their natural juices. The salt helps this process as it naturally draws out the moisture of food.

When the mixture in the bowl is covered with a small amount of liquid it is ready to be spooned into the sterilized jar.

Fill the jar, leaving a 3cm (1in) gap at the top. Use a plastic spatula to clean around the top of the jar, ensuring that the mixture is submerged under the liquid. Close the lid of the jar and leave at room temperature out of direct sunlight for 3 weeks before checking for fermentation (see page 41). When checking the mixture, use a clean spoon to taste whether the vegetables have started to ferment.

After opening, store in the refrigerator with the lid on. Fermentation will slow down at cooler temperatures and the mixture will last for up to 1 month

Borski kraut

Makes: 2 litres (3½ pints/8 cups)

800g (1lb 12oz) carrots, trimmed and peeled

800g (1lb 12oz) butternut squash

1kg (2lb 3½oz) raw beetroot (beets)

10g (½oz) caraway seeds

500g (1lb 2oz) red onion, peeled

40g (1½oz/3 tbsp) pink Himalayan salt

Put all the ingredients into a food processor (a bowl chopper). Using the pulse button, pulse until everything is roughly chopped into 1cm (½in) chunks.

Before putting them into a sterilized 2-litre (3½-pint) jar (see page 41), massage the ingredients with your hands – they should be sterilized or you can wear clean gloves – to release the natural juices.

When filling the jar, leave a 3cm (1in) gap at the top. Put the lid on securely and set aside to ferment at room temperature out of direct sunlight before opening. Check it after 3 weeks: use a clean spoon and taste to see if the vegetables have started to ferment. They will have changed colour and softened. You can eat them at this stage but the flavour will improve if you refrigerate them for longer.

After opening, store in the refrigerator with the lid on. The fermentation will slow down at cooler temperatures and will last for up to 1 month.

Thai fermented napa

Makes: 2 litres (3½ pints/8 cups)

2kg (4lb 7oz) Napa cabbage (Chinese leaf), thinly sliced

4 lemongrass stalks, peeled and finely chopped

8 dried Kaffir lime leaves

15g (½oz) fresh green chillies, deseeded and finely chopped

100g (3½oz) shallots, finely chopped

100g (3½oz) spring onions (scallions), cut into 5mm (¼in) chunks

80g (3oz) fresh root ginger, peeled and finely grated

60g (2½oz) coriander (cilantro), finely chopped

20ml (4 tsp) Thai fish sauce (nam pla)

20g (¾oz/4 tsp) good-quality sea salt

Sterilize a 2-litre (3½-pint) Kilner jar (see page 41).

Put all the ingredients in a large mixing bowl. Use a rolling pin to smash the cabbage and the other ingredients to release some of their natural juice. The salt will help as it naturally draws the moisture out of food. This will take about 5 minutes and is a great upper body workout, so go for it and get stuck in!

When the mixture in the bowl is covered with a small amount of liquid it is ready to be spooned into the sterilized jar.

Fill the jar but leave a 3cm (1in) gap at the top. Using a plastic spatula, clean around the top of the jar to ensure that all the cabbage mixture is submerged under the liquid. Close the lid and leave at room temperature out of direct sunlight for 3 weeks before checking for fermentation (see page 41). When checking the mixture, use a clean spoon to taste if the vegetables have started to ferment.

Store in the refrigerator with the lid on. The fermentation will slow down in cooler temperatures and the mixture will last for up to 1 month.

Protein-rich fasting broths

All meat stocks prepared in restaurant kitchens start with the carcass being roasted in the oven before simmering for several hours to extract the very best from the bones and marrow. The minerals that go into making up the bones are released and the resulting reduced stock is bursting with flavour and very nutrient-dense. These two fasting broths are really easy to prepare and have a complex yet delicious flavour. Enjoy these broths when you are intermittent-fasting or limiting your food intake. Both broths form the basis of many soups in the recipe section, so it is a good idea to make large amounts and batch freeze them. Never throw away a chicken carcass and buy beef bones from your butcher.

Chicken broth

This broth can be enjoyed as a soup or used as stock in other dishes throughout this book. You can make it in advance and freeze it, if wished, or you can make double or triple the quantity and then freeze for later use. To intensify the flavour, it can be reduced by one-third before adding the garnish at the end.

Serves 4

1.5kg (3lb 5oz) chicken bones
4 celery sticks
4 carrots
2 onions
5 garlic cloves
15g (½oz) coriander seeds
2 star anise
15g (½oz) fennel seeds
1 tsp Szechuan peppercorns
3 bay leaves
½ bunch of thyme
100g (3½oz/½ cup) raw minced chicken
2 egg whites

For the vegetable garnish:
2 spring onions (scallions), sliced
2.5cm (1in) fresh root ginger, peeled and cut into fine strips
thin strips of carrot
1 tsp Tamari
juice of ½ lime
pinch of chilli flakes

Preheat the oven to 200°C, 400°C, Gas mark 6.

Cut the chicken bones into small pieces. Cut the celery, carrots, onion and garlic into rough dice – approximately 2cm (¾in).

Mix the vegetables and chicken bones with the coriander seeds, star anise, fennel seeds and Szechuan peppercorns. Place them in a roasting pan and roast in the preheated oven for 30 minutes until golden brown.

Using tongs, put the roasted vegetables, chicken bones and spices into a large saucepan. Cover with 4 litres (7 pints/16 cups) cold water and then remove any visible fat from the surface of the liquid with a small spoon.

Add the bay leaves and thyme. Mix the minced chicken with the egg whites and put into the pan. Simmer very gently for at least 4 hours until reduced and well flavoured. Allow to cool and then refrigerate the broth. Strain to discard the vegetables and bones, etc.

Pour a little of the cooled broth into a 1cm (½in) deep ramekin and leave to set in the fridge to a jelly. Remove when set and cut into dice to use as part of the garnish.

Just before serving, reheat the broth and serve in bowls garnished with the chopped jelly, spring onions (scallions), ginger and carrot strips. Add the Tamari, a dash of lime juice and a few chilli flakes.

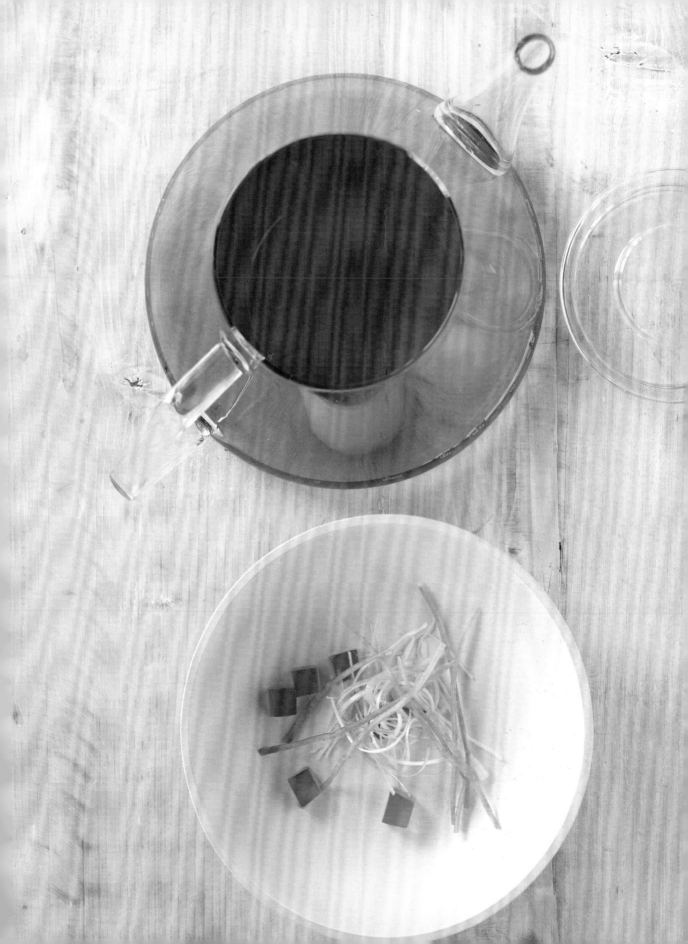

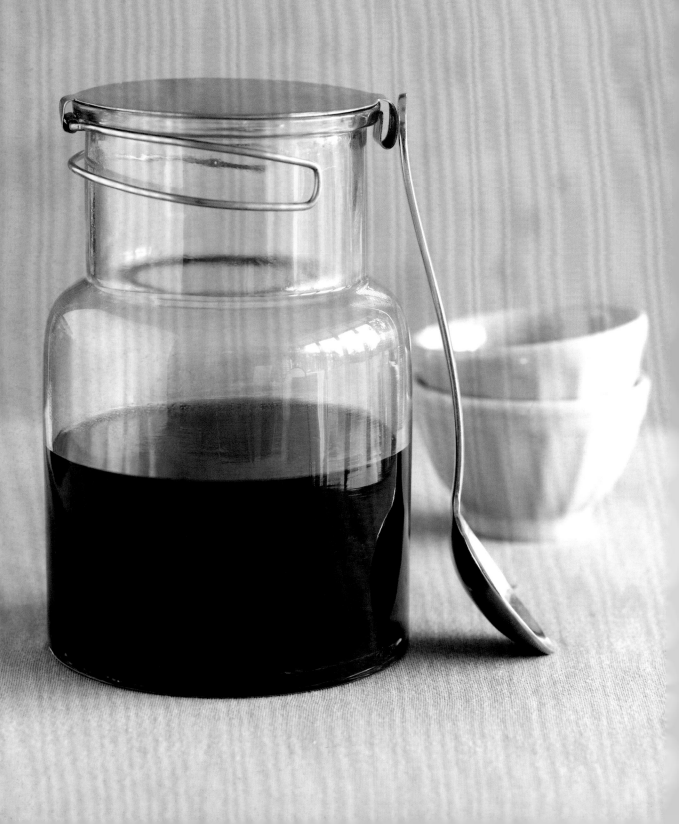

Beef broth

Nothing beats the flavour of a home-made beef broth, and, frankly, a canned consommé simply won't do, as the level of added salt is excessive. Even if you don't eat beef on a regular basis, you can purchase marrow bones from your butcher and use them to make the broth from scratch — it's worth it.

Serves 4

3kg (6lb 10oz) beef marrow bones, cut into 3cm (1in) pieces

4 carrots, chopped

3 large onions, chopped

4 celery sticks, chopped

2 bay leaves

10 whole peppercorns

½ bunch of thyme

For the garnish:

20g (¾oz) alfalfa sprouts

1 large tomato, skinned, deseeded and diced

Preheat the oven to 220°C, 425°F, Gas mark 7.

Arrange the cut marrow bones in a large roasting pan and roast in the preheated oven for 40 minutes.

Drain 2 tseaspoons of the fat from the bones into a large saucepan and sauté the vegetables over a medium heat until golden brown.

Add the bay leaves, peppercorns, sprigs of thyme and the roasted bones to the pan. Cover with 5 litres (8¾ pints/20 cups) cold water. Skim any fat from the surface and bring to a simmer. Gently cook for up to 6 hours, occasionally skimming the fat with a ladle.

Strain into another pan if reheating to eat, or into freezer trays and leave to cool before freezing. Pour a little of the broth into a 1cm (½in) deep ramekin and leave to set in the fridge to a jelly. Remove when set and chop to use as part of the garnish.

Add the garnish of chopped jelly, alfalfa sprouts and diced tomato to the hot broth just before serving.

NUTRITION FACTS

Beef marrow bones yield one of the highest sources of all nine essential amino acids for healing, repair and rebuilding every cell in the body. Together with the B vitamins magnesium and potassium from the vegetables, they provide everything the body needs during a period of limited food intake.

Heal yourself with the 21-day plan

We recommend following the Plan for at least three weeks to ensure that your digestive tract gets the rest and repair it needs. The results, over this period of time, can really be substantial and it is worth making the commitment to following it. When your symptoms have improved within that time, producing more energy, improved skin, hair, and nails (and a flatter tummy), it will be easier to repeat the Plan on a bi-annual or quarterly basis for maximum impact.

MAKING THE PLAN WORK FOR YOU

Here are some basic guidelines to help you to follow the Plan and adapt it to your daily routine and lifestyle.

- Plan your meals and shopping lists in advance when you have time to avoid 'panic' buying and eating.
- Have 'cooking sessions' – at weekends or evenings – to prepare fresh food, e.g. blanching salad ingredients. Wash and store the ingredients either in sealed plastic containers or zip-lock bags to keep them fresh and crisp in the fridge for quick assembly later.
- Make up sufficient broths for fasting evenings. These can be frozen if you're making up large batches – split them into 300ml (½-pint) quantities and seal in small containers, remembering to label them with the date and name to avoid confusion.
- You may swap the meals around to suit your plans for a particular day, but make sure you always have a substantial percentage of protein with each meal (approximately 50 per cent) to provide the healing and repairing amino acids found in such foods.
- Remember to start each main meal with one of the sauerkrauts and a dose of bitters to increase the efficacy of your stomach acids and digestive enzymes. Either make your own from the recipes provided, or buy the commercially-produced versions.
- Eating *light at night* is best for your digestion – and for regulating blood sugar levels. Many people have their main meal in the evening, then wake up in the middle of the night as their digestion struggles to cope with the overload. Eating light also helps to relieve heartburn and indigestion during the night.

- Prepare dishes in the evening to take with you to work the following day; store in containers ready to grab-and-go in the morning. Choose foods that will not perish en route. Alternatively, cook extra for the evening meal and keep some of the prepared dish as part of your meal following lunchtime, with added salad and/or soup.
- Make up bottles of different salad dressings to keep in the fridge. You can purchase small squeezy cosmetic bottles to transport these to your workplace.
- Eating out need never be difficult or challenging provided that you follow the principles of the Plan and choose restaurants that are able to serve good-quality poultry and fish and plenty of green vegetables on the side – remember, puddings are out!
- If travelling, make sure you have prepared easy-to-transport meals, such as almond and coconut pancakes, spinach butternut squash and lentil frittata, butter bean hummus, or any of the salads that you can make up in advance and take with you. Remember that liquids can't be taken on aeroplanes, so soups and smoothies are out.

A 14-DAY MEAL PLANNER

The 14-day meal planner opposite has been devised only as a guide to give you an idea of the dishes you can eat on a daily basis on the Plan and the variety you need to ensure maximum nutritional benefit. Whilst we encourage you to eat light at night, you may want to consume quality protein and vegetables with your evening meal, reserving some of that meal for part of your lunch the next day. Soups, hot or cold, can easily be transported in a thermos flask for ease at work.

A 14-DAY MEAL PLANNER

	BREAKFAST	LUNCH	SUPPER
DAY 1	Chia muesli Ginger and lemon herbal tea	Shiitake, bean & fennel soup Spinach, butternut & lentil frittata	Shredded pheasant salad with pickled mushrooms Slow-roasted peppers & aubergines
DAY 2	Maca, avocado, pear, apple and mint smoothie Herbal tea	Marinated grilled chicken breast Butterbean hummus with tomato & avocado salsa	Fasting – Beef broth only
DAY 3	Fasting – herbal teas only	Lamb koftas Roasted cauliflower ratatouille	Shiitake, bean and fennel soup Grilled asparagus & poached egg
DAY 4	Baked eggs with tomato, pepper & chorizo Peppermint tea	Red lentil & lemon soup, no Chermoula Sardine fillets with green beans, red onions & olives	Lamb with grilled asparagus and salsa verde Purple sprouting broccoli with brazil nuts, sesame & orange
DAY 5	Asian-style salmon tartar on chia wasabi crackers Green tea	Cold lamb cutlets Salad 3 with dressing of choice	Fasting – Chicken broth only
DAY 6	Fasting – Herbal teas only	Pea, broad been & lovage velouté Spiced chicken burgers Salad 1 with dressing of choice	Red pepper, tomato, date & lime soup Escabeche of red mullet Pak choy with lentils & lime
DAY 7	Ful medames with poached eggs Herbal tea	Red pepper, tomato, date & lime soup Pak Choy with lentils & lime Salad 2 with dressing of choice	Roasted tamarind, chilli, ginger & coriander chicken Roasted beetroot with chipotle
DAY 8	Chia, poppy seed & lime muffins with raspberry purée Herbal tea	Shredded tamarind chicken Salad 2 with dressing of choice plus added vegetables of choice	Marinated rib-eye of beef (no sweet potato!) Grilled baby leeks with romesco plus added vegetables of choice
DAY 9	Almond & coconut pancakes with roasted spiced plums Herbal tea	Marinated grilled chicken breast with paprika Green beans with hazelnut & pea pesto	Fasting – Beef broth only
DAY 10	Fasting – Herbal teas only	Moroccan spiced pumpkin soup Marinated rib-eye of beef (no sweet potato!) Salad 4 with dressing of choice	Grilled sole fillets marinated in ginger & tangerine juice Purple sprouting broccoli
DAY 11	Baked eggs with tomato, pepper & chorizo Lemon or white tea	Smokey aubergine soup Cold sole fillet (leftover from supper) Salad 1 with dressing of choice	Chicken livers with apple, pancetta & shallots Cauliflower ratatouille
DAY 12	Summer fruits en papillote Macadamia & berry smoothie	Spinach, butternut & lentil frittata Pak choy with lentils & lime	Fasting – Chicken broth only
DAY 13	Fasting – Herbal teas only	Shiitake, bean & fennel soup Tomato & avocado salsa Shredded pheasant salad	Fillet of pork Purple sprouting broccoli Grilled baby leeks with romesco
DAY 14	Ful medames White or green tea	Broccoli, avocado, almond & mint soup Spiced chicken burgers Salad 2 with dressing of choice	Marinated grilled mackerel with fennel Roasted cherry tomatoes with maple syrup & chilli Steamed vegetables of choice

Taking it further

The beauty of this Plan is that it is designed to be sustainable, improving your health and, by default, offering you a better way to eat. Having put so much effort into changing your diet over the last three weeks or so, you should now be feeling the benefits of eating well and realizing it is key to substantially better health. The modifications you've already made have gone a long way to helping your body repair itself through improved digestive function.

TAKE STOCK OF YOUR HEALTH

Once any symptoms of poor health have abated, your health and energy have improved and your digestion is functioning optimally, you can extend the list of foods you can eat. In order to move on, you must embrace any major changes that have been proven to work unequivocally for you – if quitting all dairy has left you feeling better with greatly improved digestion, no more headaches and improved skin, then reintroducing small amounts of goat's and sheep's cheeses (which are less likely to produce inflammation than cow's dairy) may be fine, but only on an occasional basis, rather than daily. Similarly, if grains (especially those that include gluten, such as wheat, oats, rye and barley) prove to be irritating or cause fatigue, there are others you can introduce at this stage, without any fuss or complications, thanks to the recipes in this book. You will need to determine what has made the most significant difference to your health. Taking stock of how it has improved over the last few weeks will motivate you to take it further.

PROTEIN IS PARAMOUNT

The importance of eating some protein with every meal cannot be over-estimated. This helps to balance blood sugar levels, so you shouldn't experience any unnecessary cravings, or peaks and troughs in energy that might lead to a tempting 'quick fix'. Eating your favourite proteins and making sure your fridge is always well stocked are the best ways to help you stay on track and to eat regularly and in balance throughout the day.

What you are aiming to achieve is providing your digestion with great-quality proteins for healing and

repair at every meal, combined with lightly cooked vegetables and fruit that maintain the supply of essential nutrients and antioxidants you need on a daily basis to support your body's natural functions. Together with some whole grains, the salads and vegetables supply the minerals that are vital for good health, as well as fibre to help transport the food and subsequently clear away any waste matter through the digestive tract efficiently. These are essential components for success post-Plan. As before, on the Plan, eating seasonal food provides variety, and sourcing the best-quality livestock, poultry and seafood pays enormous dividends in the quality of the nutrients they deliver.

INTERMITTENT FASTING

Intermittent fasting is the silent key to unlocking the door to your health. Just as we rest when we sleep, so our digestion needs a break periodically to readjust and revitalize its own function. We strongly recommend that you continue this practice, if only once a week, as the medical benefits are now scientifically proven, and millions of people are experiencing better health due to choosing this means of periodic food restriction.

POST-PLAN ALLOWED GRAINS

Having cut out all grains during the Plan, owing to the gluten in the most common ones (wheat, oats, rye and barley) being potentially irritating to the intestinal lining, and removing the types of carbohydrates that the body may find difficult to completely break down, at this stage you can include some of the alternative grains that nourish your body, without taxing your digestive system. Soaking grains overnight with added citrus juice, such as lemon or lime juice, inhibits the phytates and enzyme inhibitors that can bind to minerals and prevent them from being absorbed. It also activates the enzymes within the grains, yielding a higher level of nutrients than when they are cooked from dry. Always rinse thoroughly before cooking further.

Buckwheat This grain provides abundant B vitamins for energy production at a cellular level, rutin for cardiovascular health and supporting the strength of micro-capillaries in the brain, zinc for boosting the immune system, and calcium and magnesium for strong bones and a healthy heart.

Jumbo oats Oats have the lowest gluten content of all the gluten-grains; you can now buy steel-cut jumbo oats with their gluten removed, allowing for the occasional muesli, porridge and topping for fruit crumbles. Oats are rich in calcium and magnesium for a healthy heart and nervous system, zinc to support immunity and B vitamins to enhance energy production.

Amaranth This lesser-known grain has the benefit of being small in structure, making it excellent for coating fish, chicken and seafood and adding energy and fibre. It is rich in calcium, magnesium, iron and the amino acid L-Lysine which has potent anti-viral properties. It's good for heart and bone health, and immunity.

Quinoa Strictly speaking, quinoa is not a real grain but it is cooked and eaten in a similar way. It's a rich source of B vitamins for energy, magnesium, manganese, folate and zinc, and it's good for bone and ligament strength, hair, skin and nails. The essential fats and phytonutrients provide an anti-inflammatory alternative to grains in sensitive people with a history of inflammatory bowel disease. Cook it in the same way as rice.

Bulghur wheat Most couscous is made from bulghur wheat, which is the whole-grain version of wheat, with its hull still intact. It provides abundant iron and B6, which helps to regulate mood and concentration.

Spelt Far lower in gluten than conventional wheat, spelt is perfect for people who tend to be intolerant to wheat. It contains calcium, magnesium, folic acid, zinc and beta-carotene as well as fibre and antioxidant-rich nutrients. It's good for the heart and nervous system.

DAIRY

If lactose-intolerance was identified during your first three to four weeks on the Plan, it's better not to re-introduce any dairy at all but instead to use nut and grain alternatives, such as coconut, almond, hazelnut, amaranth, quinoa or brown rice milks. However, make sure that no sugar has been added to any of these. Do not be tempted by soya milks as so many are made from genetically-modified soya beans, which is not a whole-food method of growing the beans. Alternatively, make these nut or grain milks yourself, as they will always taste better and will be richer in nutrients, too.

If you've never had any problems with cow's, sheep's or goat's milk or their produce, you can choose an

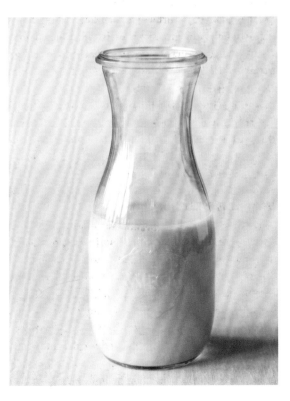

organic variety, buying whole milk, cream and crème fraiche. Don't be tempted to buy the low-fat versions of any of these foods, as lowering their fat removes the CLA (conjugated linoleic acid) that is responsible for helping to burn the fat stored around your torso, arms and legs. Nor should you ever buy homogenized dairy as this process removes many of the nutrients that are an essential part of the protein.

Yoghurt Home-made 24-hour fermented yoghurt has absorbed the lactose in milk (see the recipe below) and allows for natural production of beneficial bacteria. You can use this yoghurt in breakfast dishes or as an accompaniment to fruit. This is infinitely preferable to commercially produced pasteurized yoghurts, which have very little or no probiotics (micro-organisms that provide us with health benefits when eaten) at all.

Cheese Seek out artisan cheeses at local farmers' markets and specialist delis. Do not buy mass-produced cheeses that are wrapped in plastic and laced with abundant preservatives and additives.

Goat's cheese Goat's milk has an essential fatty acid profile that is similar to human breast milk and it is tolerated well by some people who cannot eat cow's dairy. Try introducing small amounts to start with to avoid a reoccurrence of related symptoms. This cheese is a good source of vitamin A and choline, which are important for eye health, and calcium and iron for a healthy heart and energy.

PEAS, LENTILS AND PULSES
On the Plan, pulses are limited to split peas, lentils, haricot and butter (lima) beans, as these are easier to break down, resulting in a small amount of protein and monosaccharides. Because their breakdown is incomplete, they feed the pathogenic bacteria in the digestive system. Post-Plan, you can widen this group to include a highly nutritious group of vegetable-based proteins (opposite). These are all excellent for lowering your cholesterol, regulating blood sugar levels, and providing slow-release energy. If using canned beans and pulses, make sure you rinse them thoroughly before adding to dishes such as soups and casseroles.

24-hour fermented yoghurt

Makes: 950ml (1 pint 12fl oz/4 cups)
950ml (1 pint 12fl oz/4 cups) full-fat cow's or goat's milk
65g (2½fl oz/¼ cup) plain yoghurt with live cultures

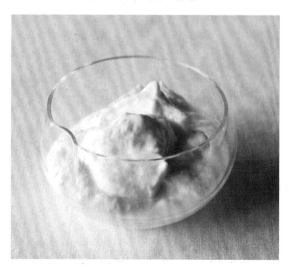

Put the milk in a heavy-based saucepan over a medium to low heat. Using a sugar thermometer, heat the milk, stirring occasionally, to 82°C, 180°F. If you don't have a thermometer, look for small bubbles forming around the edge of the pan.

Remove the pan from the heat and set aside to cool until the milk reaches room temperature. If you add the starter to milk that's too hot, you'll kill it.

Blend 125ml (4fl oz/½ cup)of cooled milk with the yoghurt in a separate bowl. Mix this into the remaining cooled milk.

Pour into clean sterilized glass bottles or a glass jar and cover with cling film (plastic wrap). Place in the oven (turn the light on inside without heating the oven, so it's approximately 38°C, 100°F) and leave to ferment for 24 hours. By this time, the lactose should be completely digested.

Allow to cool to room temperature before storing the yoghurt in the fridge.

Note: When it comes out of the oven it may still be runny, but it will solidify as it cools.

A 7-DAY POST-PLAN MEAL PLANNER

	BREAKFAST	LUNCH	SUPPER
DAY 1	Winter/Summer Bircher-style muesli Green tea	Moroccan spiced pumpkin soup Spinach, butternut & lentil frittata	Grilled sole fillets in ginger & tangerine juice Sweet potato salad with mango & apricot
DAY 2	Peach & vanilla smoothie with frozen raspberry yoghurt	Marinated grilled chicken breast with slow-roasted peppers, aubergines, anchovies & almonds	**Fasting** – Beef broth only
DAY 3	**Fasting** – Herbal teas only	Red lentil, apricot & preserved lemon soup Lamb kofta with green beans & hazelnut & pea pesto	Sweet potato & chickpea cakes Roasted cauliflower ratatouille
DAY 4	Baked eggs with tomato, peppers & chorizo Peppermint tea	Shiitake bean & fennel soup Butterbean hummus with tomato & avocado salsa, quinoa flatbreads	Lamb cutlets with grilled asparagus & salsa verde Jerk spiced roast butternut squash
DAY 5	Pumpkin pancakes with crispy pancetta Ginger and lemon tea	Cold lamb cutlets Salad 3 with dressing of choice	**Fasting** – Chicken broth only
DAY 6	**Fasting** – Herbal teas only	Spiced coconut & roasted carrot soup Crispy strips of amaranth chicken with roasted beetroot, chipotle & tangerines	Confit of salmon with bulgur salad Pak choy with lentils & lime
DAY 7	Savoury goat's cheese flapjack Lemongrass tea	Beef carpaccio with pepper, chilli & ginger Salad 1 with dressing of choice	Pan-fried calves' liver with butter bean and sage purée Roasted pumpkin with chilli, cashews & lemon

Chickpeas These are great for a snack, as in falafels, or salads as they are packed with healthy minerals that reduce the damaging LDL cholesterol (collects in the walls of blood vessels) and help balance blood sugar levels. They are full of manganese, copper, iron and zinc.

Borlotti beans Rich in vitamin B1 and iron for energy, borlotti beans are good for regulating blood sugar levels and help you to stay feeling fuller for longer.

ADDITIONAL VEGETABLES

In addition to some dairy, whole grains and beans, you can also start extending your repertoire of vegetables post-Plan to include more roots as well as squashes.

Butternut squash Full of B vitamins, vitamin K, beta-carotene and magnesium, these winter squash deliver plenty of energy, natural sweetness and a starchy texture without upsetting your blood sugar levels.

Parsnip Rich in vitamin C, folic acid and fibre, parsnips are often thought of as a high GI (glycaemic index) food, disrupting blood sugar levels. However, they are a great high-fibre alternative to potatoes, being lower in starch.

Sweet potato One of the best naturally sweet root vegetables, sweet potato is rich in beta-carotene and vitamin C as well as all the B vitamins, providing slow-release energy and helping to balance your mood.

Jerusalem artichokes An abundant source of iron, copper and vitamin C, they are great for hair health and as good a source of potassium as bananas for regulating cardiovascular health and blood pressure.

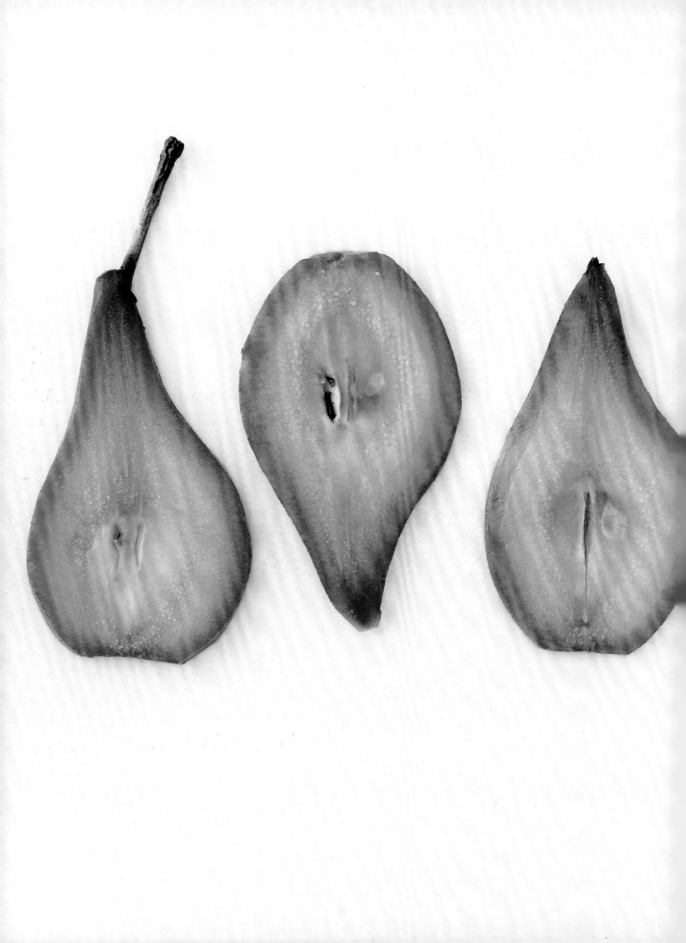

Breakfasts

(P) Summer fruit en papillote

This a beautiful way of presenting lightly steamed seasonal fruits, with vanilla, cinnamon and a hint of aniseed to enliven them. Wrapped individually for maximum impact, the aromas are revealed on opening, whilst the nutritional value is preserved.

Serves 4

4 pineapple slices, peeled, cored and sliced

8 strawberries, hulled and halved

16 raspberries

handful of blackberries

1 vanilla pod (bean), cut into 4 pieces

2 cinnamon sticks, halved

4 whole star anise

4 thick strips of zest, cut from 1 orange with a potato peeler

For the blackcurrant sauce:

1 punnet of blackcurrants

5 tsp local runny honey

Preheat the oven to 200°C, 400°F, Gas mark 6.

Make the blackcurrant sauce: wash the blackcurrants and put them in a small stainless steel pan with the honey. Bring to a simmer and cook gently for 5 minutes. Remove from the heat and allow to cool.

To prepare the papillote, cut out 4 large squares of parchment paper, 30 x 30cm (12 x 12in) and fold each one over diagonally to form a triangle. Open up again to form a square and drizzle 2 tablespoons of blackcurrant sauce along the crease in the middle. Neatly arrange the fruit on top of the sauce. Arrange the vanilla pod (bean), cinnamon sticks, star anise and orange zest on top of the fruit (so they can be removed easily before eating).

Fold over the paper to make a triangle and then crimp the edges to form an airtight seal. Place each triangular package carefully on a flat baking sheet ready to cook.

Cook in the preheated oven for 10 minutes, until the packages are puffed up and full of steam.

Serve the fruit packages immediately, ready to be opened at the table using a sharp knife.

CHEF'S TIP

These delicious fruit parcels can also be cooked on the barbecue. Simply place the parchment parcels on a square of silver foil, to transfer the heat from the hot coals through to the parcel.

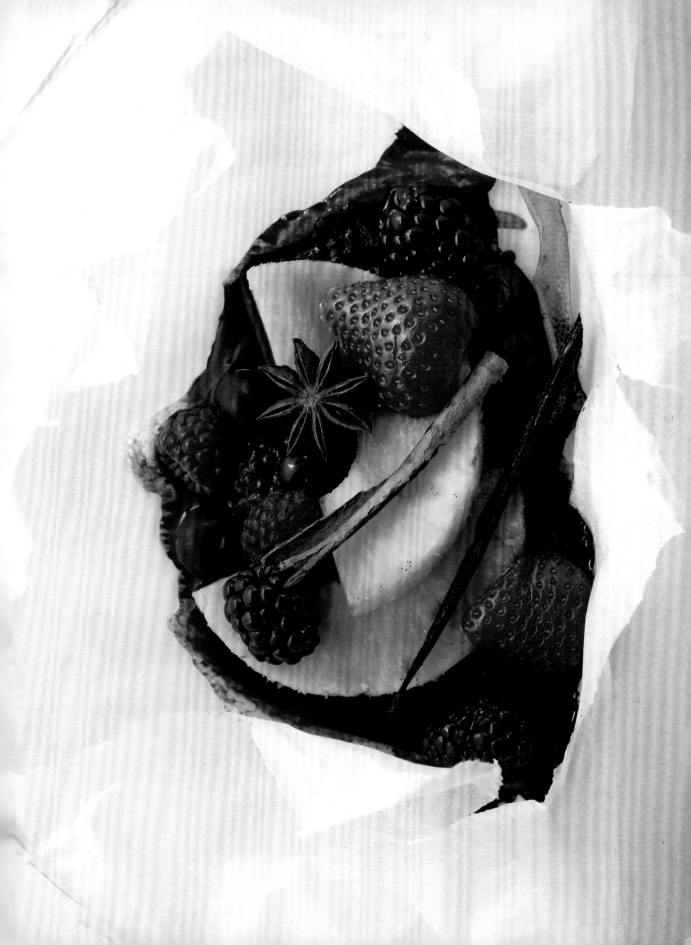

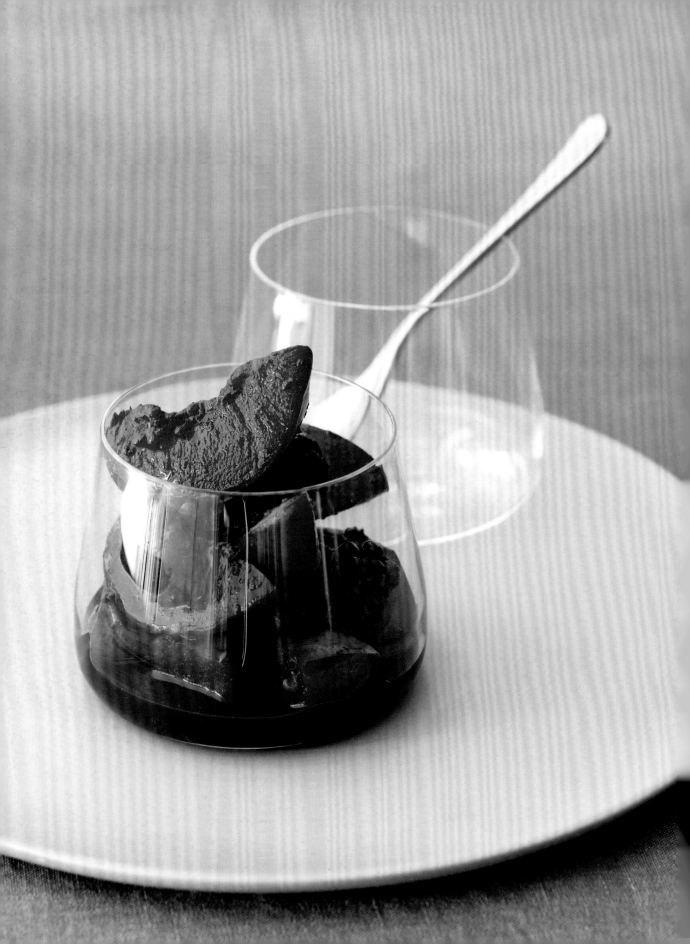

P Autumn apple, pear and plum compôte

Poaching fruits softens their fibre, thereby enabling easier digestion, which conforms with the principles of the Plan. Use locally bought seasonal apples, pears and plums. Adding soaked nuts provides this dish with the correct balance of protein and essential fatty acids.

Serves 4

200g (7oz) red Braeburn or Cox's apples, cored and diced

200g (7oz) green Granny Smith's apple, cored and diced

150g (5oz) Conference pears, cored and cut into 8 wedges

150g (5oz) plums, stoned and cut into 6 pieces

100g (3½oz/scant ⅓ cup) blackberries, fresh or frozen

50g (2oz/⅓ cup) macadamia nuts, soaked in water overnight

50g (2oz/⅓ cup) cashew nuts, soaked in water overnight

50g (2oz/⅓ cup) whole peeled almonds, soaked in water overnight

For the syrup:

400ml (14fl oz/1⅔ cups) water

4 star anise

5 green cardamom pods

1 tsp ground cinnamon

2 whole bay leaves

1 tsp finely grated orange zest

6 tbsp apple juice

2 tbsp local runny honey

To make the syrup, put all the ingredients in a steel saucepan and simmer gently, uncovered, over a low heat until the syrup has reduced by half.

Add the apples and simmer for 5 minutes, then add the pears, plums and blackberries, and simmer for a further 5 minutes. Remove from the heat and allow to cool in the liquid before storing in an airtight container in the refrigerator for up to 4 days.

To serve, decant the fruit onto serving plates. Serve with a little of the syrup and a sprinkle of soaked nuts (if wished), which have been rinsed under cold running water and dried on kitchen paper.

VARIATION

Other fruits can be used for this dish. The above fruits are great in the autumn, but other seasonal fruits can be substituted. Try using blackcurrants, instead of blackberries, with summer fruits.

NUTRITION FACTS

The blackberries in this recipe provide an abundance of beta-carotene and vitamin C to boost immunity, as well as zinc from the nuts.

P Exotic fruit soup with ginger & lime

The combination of spicy coconut milk and delicate fresh fruits is a surprise to the palate. Packed with antioxidant vitamins and beta-carotene, the fruits protect the digestion, whilst papaya is packed with naturally-occurring enzymes to help break down the food.

Serves 4

400ml (14fl oz/1⅔ cups) coconut milk

30g (1oz) lemongrass stalks, peeled and chopped

30g (1oz) fresh root ginger, peeled and roughly chopped

2 kaffir lime leaves

20ml (4 tsp) lime juice

grated zest of ½ lime

4 tsp local runny honey

100g (3½oz) watermelon, peeled and cut into 2cm (1in) chunks

8 lychees, peeled, stoned and quartered

1 papaya, skinned, deseeded and cut into 2cm (1in) chunks

8 fresh mint leaves, finely shredded

To make the coconut soup, blitz the coconut milk, lemongrass, ginger, kaffir lime leaves, lime juice and zest, and honey in a blender – or use a hand blender. Leave in a covered container in the fridge for 1 hour before passing through a fine sieve ready to serve.

Divide the prepared fruits between 4 soup plates. Using a whisk, beat the chilled coconut soup until it froths slightly and pour it over the fruits.

Serve immediately, garnished with shredded mint.

NUTRITION FACTS

Watermelon has a very high level of potassium, which helps to balance excess sodium in the body. It is low in sugar and, unlike other melons, it's protected from developing mould spores owing to the thick skin.

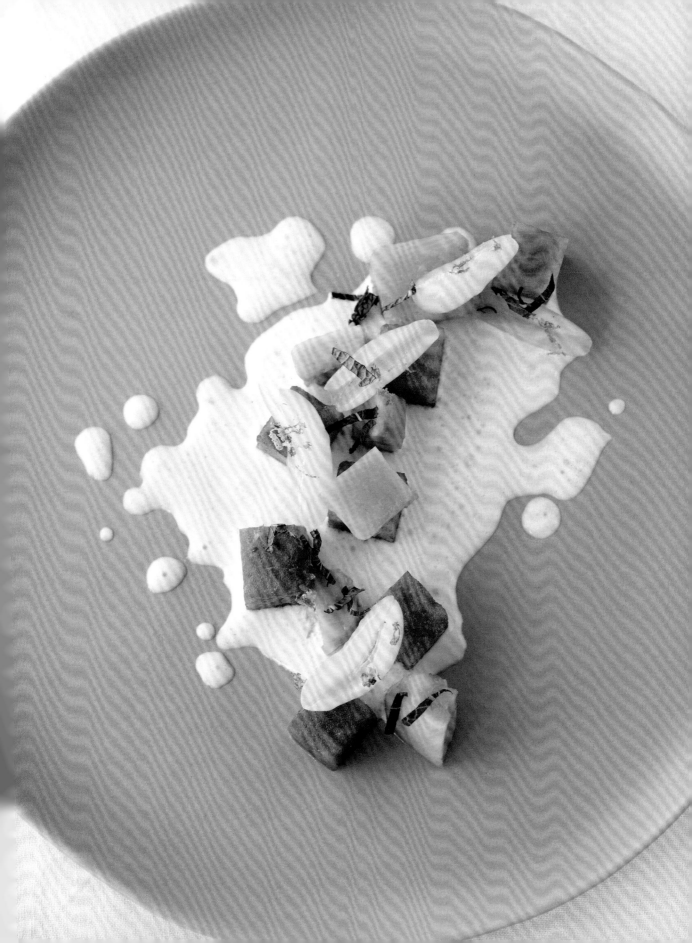

P Maca, avocado, pear, apple & mint smoothie

This protein-packed morning smoothie is full of skin-nourishing nutrients and has a potent malty, caramel flavour. It can be put in a sealed container and taken to work for breakfast, or even frozen into individual lollies for eating as nutritious summer treats.

Makes 1 litre (1¾ pints/4 cups)

850ml (1⅓ pints/3½ cups) unsweetened almond milk

100g (3½oz) pear, peeled and cored

100g (3½oz) apple, peeled and cored

150g (5oz) avocado, peeled and stoned

10g (½oz) fresh mint leaves

15g (½oz) maca powder

juice of ½ lime

Make sure that all the ingredients are thoroughly chilled before blending. Using a jug blender, blitz all the ingredients until smooth. Serve the smoothie in chilled glasses over ice.

Note: This smoothie keeps well in the fridge overnight in an airtight container.

P Macadamia & berry smoothie

A rich source of antioxidant berries, combined with the essential fats, zinc and magnesium of the macadamia nuts, this smoothie is balanced in flavour and provides a satisfying alternative to a solid food breakfast. It's also great on-the-run or as a pre-workout drink.

Makes 1 litre (1¾ pints/4 cups)

100g (3½oz/scant ½ cup) blackberries, fresh or frozen

100g (3½oz/1 cup) strawberries, hulled

100g (3½oz/¾ cup) raspberries, fresh or frozen

150g (5oz/1 cup) macadamia nuts, soaked overnight

200g (7oz) mango, peeled and stoned

700ml (1 pint 3½fl oz/scant 3 cups) coconut water

seeds of ½ vanilla pod (bean)

acai powder, for dusting

Lay the fresh blackberries, strawberries and raspberries on a tray and freeze overnight.

Strain the macadamia nuts. In a large jug blender, blitz all the ingredients, except the acai powder, until smooth. Serve in chilled glasses with a sprinkling of acai powder.

Note: This smoothie keeps well in the fridge overnight in an airtight container.

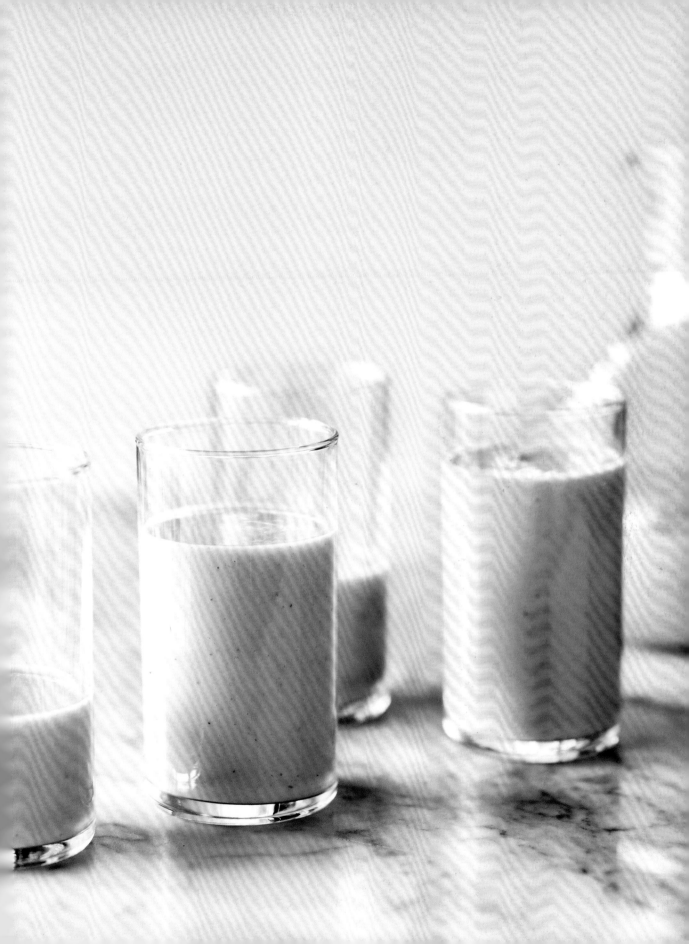

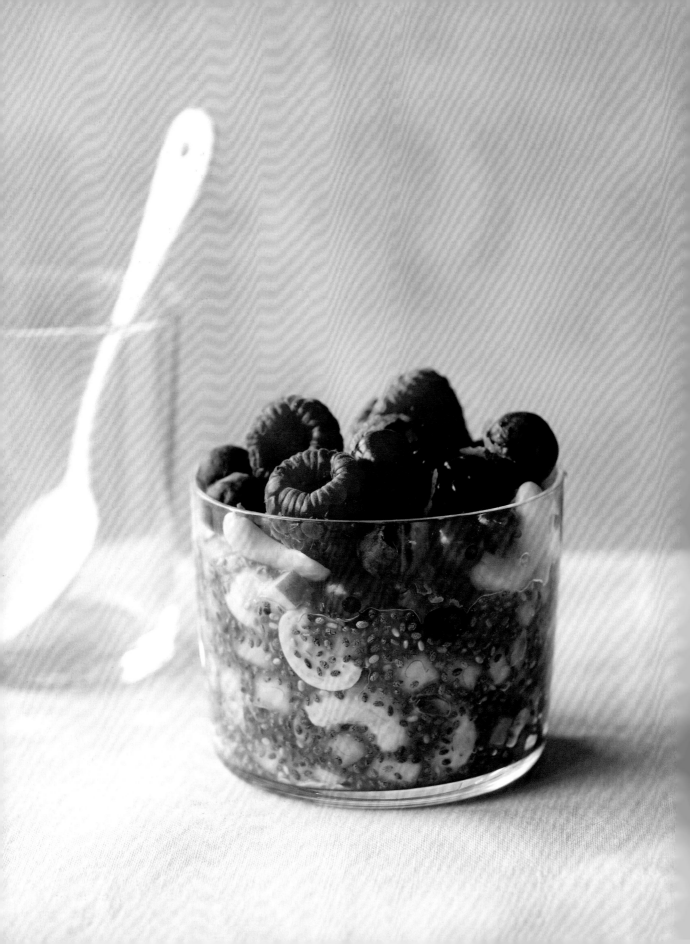

(P) Chia muesli

A satisfying gluten-free alternative to the traditional oat-based muesli. Chia is the seed of the chia grain and a real superfood. Light yet satisfying, the combination of protein from the soaked chia and cashews, mixed with the antioxidant-rich berries creates a 'pudding-style' breakfast.

Serves 4

70g (2¾oz) chia seeds

½ tsp mixed spice

2 tsp local runny honey

300ml (½ pint/1¼ cups) water

200g (7oz) red apples, skin on, cored and cut into 5mm (¼in) dice

150g (5oz) pears, skin on, cored and cut into 5mm (¼in) dice

100g (3½oz) cashew nuts, soaked in water overnight

24 blueberries

12 raspberries

2 strawberries, halved

orange zest for the topping

In a bowl, mix together the chia seeds, mixed spice, honey and water. Whisk and then rest for 5 minutes.

Mix the diced apples and pears with the cashews, and then combine with the chia mixture. Divide between 4 glasses and top with the blueberries, raspberries, strawberries and orange zest.

NUTRITION FACTS

Chia seeds absorb up to 17 times their weight in fluids, swelling to create an Omega-3 packed food that does not irritate the gut. It has vegetable-based protein and more calcium and iron than milk or spinach.

P Almond & coconut pancakes with roasted spiced plums

These delicious protein-rich pancakes can be cooked by the dozen and frozen successfully. Almond and coconut flours provide a grain-free alternative, as per the principles of the Plan, as well as abundant minerals and vitamins for boosting energy at the start of the day.

Serves 4

For the pancakes:
100g (3½oz/scant ¾ cup) ground almonds
25g (1oz/⅛ cup) coconut flour
1 tsp ground cinnamon
1½ tsp baking powder (baking soda)
4 organic free-range eggs
200ml (7fl oz/generous ¾ cup) coconut milk
seeds from 1 vanilla pod (bean)
1 tbsp local runny honey
2 tbsp coconut oil

For the plums:
12 ripe plums
1 tbsp local runny honey
1 tsp mixed spice
1 tsp grated orange zest
2 tbsp orange juice

Preheat the oven to 200°C, 400°F, Gas mark 6.

Cut the plums in half, discarding the stones, and place 8 of them, cut-side up, on a parchment-lined baking sheet. Mix together the honey, mixed spice, orange zest and juice and pour over the plums. Roast for 15 minutes in the oven, then remove and allow to cool. As the plums cool, they will release their natural juice.

Blend the remaining 4 plums with the cooking juices and set aside.

To make the pancakes, put the ground almonds in a large mixing bowl. Sift the coconut flour, cinnamon and baking powder (baking soda) over the top and mix together thoroughly.

In a separate bowl, whisk the eggs with the coconut milk, vanilla seeds and honey, and then beat this into the dry mixture to make a smooth batter.

Heat a small non-stick frying pan over a low heat. Add a little coconut oil and drop a large spoonful of pancake batter into the hot pan (the mixture should be enough for 4 pancakes). Cook for 1 minute, then flip the pancake over and cook for a further minute on the other side until golden brown. Slide out of the pan and keep warm while you cook the remaining pancakes in the same way.

Reheat the plums gently. Serve the pancakes with the warm plums, drizzled with the plum sauce made from the juices.

NUTRITION FACTS

Coconut is rich in Omega-nutrition that does not spoil easily when heated, whilst almonds provide plenty of magnesium to calm the mind as well as the gut.

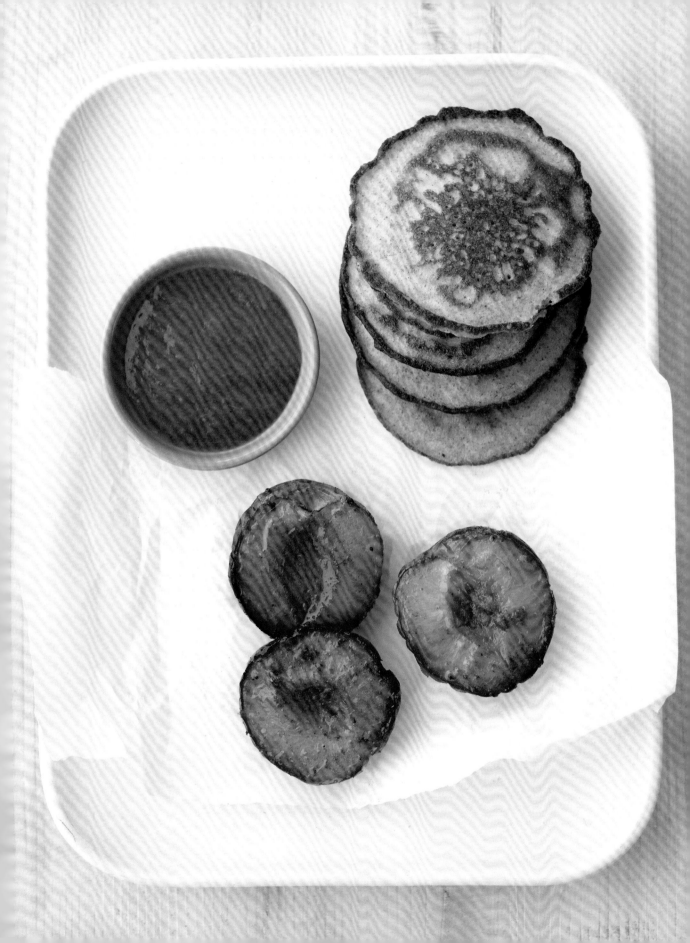

Ⓟ Pumpkin pancakes with crispy pancetta & green tomato

Although seemingly complex, these protein-rich pancakes are divine, and making the batter is well worth the effort. Why not make your own lentil flour in a spice grinder? It can be tricky to find, and you can store it in a container in the fridge. The pancakes may be batch cooked and frozen.

Serves 4

12 rashers thinly sliced pancetta (see opposite)

150g (5oz) pumpkin, skinned, deseeded and cut into 1cm (½in) dice

100g (3½oz) pine nuts (pignoli), soaked overnight

3 large organic free-range eggs

½ tsp ground coriander

½ tsp ground cumin

½ tsp ground turmeric

pinch of sea salt

50g (2oz/⅓ cup) red lentil flour

1 tsp baking powder (baking soda)
50g (2oz) clarified butter

4 green tomatoes, quartered and pan-fried in a little clarified butter

Arrange the pancetta rashers on a non-stick baking tray ready for cooking. Preheat the oven to 170°C, 325°F, Gas mark 3.

Put the diced pumpkin in an ovenproof dish and roast in the preheated oven for about 20 minutes, until soft. Remove and allow to cool.

Put the pumpkin in a food processor and blend until smooth. Add the pine nuts (pignoli), eggs, coriander, cumin and turmeric. Blend together before adding the salt, lentil flour and baking powder (baking soda). Transfer the pancake batter to a bowl, cover and keep in the fridge until ready to cook.

Cook the pancetta in the preheated oven until crisp, or cook under the grill. Drain on kitchen paper and keep warm.

To make the pancakes, heat a little of the clarified butter in a pan over a low heat and spoon dessertspoons of the batter into the pan. Cook for about 1½ minutes on each side, until set and golden brown. You should have enough batter for 8 pancakes.

Place 2 pancakes on each serving plate and serve with the crispy pancetta and pan-fried green tomatoes.

Note: Use aluminium and gluten-free baking powder. Make your own by mixing together 1 tsp bicarbonate of soda (baking soda), 2 tsp cream of tartar and 1 tsp arrowroot in a bowl. Store in a small airtight container.

NUTRITION FACTS

Organic or grass-fed pork is richer in Omega-3 and vitamin E than its farmed equivalent, as the pigs forage on wild foods rather than commercial grains. Making pancetta this way (see opposite) is infinitely preferable as it contains none of the nitrates in packaged bacon and ham.

(P) Home-made pancetta

Makes 1.5kg (3lb 5oz) finished pancetta

20g (¾oz) juniper berries

10 bay leaves

20g (¾oz) fennel seeds

15g (½oz) black peppercorns

1 whole nutmeg, grated

60g (2¼oz) sea salt

15g (½oz) fresh rosemary leaves, chopped

15g (½oz) fresh thyme leaves

6 garlic cloves, grated

3 tbsp maple syrup

2kg (4½lb) pork belly, boned and skinned

Using a herb grinder or pestle and mortar, grind the juniper berries, bay leaves, fennel seeds and black peppercorns. Transfer to a bowl and add the grated nutmeg, salt, herbs and garlic. Add the maple syrup and mix thoroughly.

Lay a large piece of cling film (plastic wrap) on a work surface and place the pork on top. Rub half the spice mixture into the skin side of the pork and the remainder into the rib side. Massage thoroughly, making sure that the dry cure mix is rubbed well into the pork.

Wrap the pork tightly in the cling film (plastic wrap) and then add a few extra layers of cling film. Place it in a deep tray that will fit in the fridge. Place a heavy weigh on top, such as a chopping board weighted down with a 4kg (9lb) weight. Leave in the fridge for 7 days, turning the pork over once every day.

After 7 days, remove the cling film. Thoroughly wash off the dry cure mix under running cold water and then pat dry with kitchen paper. Place the pork on a wooden board and keep in the fridge, uncovered, for 2 weeks, turning it once every 2 days. After this time you will have delicious pancetta ready for slicing thinly before cooking.

ⓟ Baked eggs with tomatoes, peppers & chorizo

Prepare the sauce the night before to give you a head-start in the morning. This may be batch-cooked and frozen successfully. It is perfect when you need a full meal in the morning, but it can also be eaten as a light supper as it fulfills all the principles of the Plan.

Serves 4

1 green (bell) pepper
12 slices chorizo cooking sausage
100g (3½oz) onion, sliced
1 garlic clove, sliced
250g (8oz/1 cup) canned chopped tomatoes
1 tsp fresh thyme, chopped
1 tsp paprika
pinch of chilli powder
150ml (¼ pint/⅔ cup) chicken stock
1 tsp coconut palm sugar
pinch of salt
4 organic free-range eggs
chopped parsley, to garnish
drizzle of olive oil

Preheat the oven to 170°C, 325°F, Gas mark 3.

Roast the green (bell) pepper in the preheated oven for 20 minutes. When the skin is blistered, allow to cool, then peel, core, deseed and shred into fine strips.

Over a low heat, cook the chorizo in a pan until the fat is released, then add the onion and fry over a medium heat until golden brown. Add the garlic and cook for 2 minutes. Reduce the heat and add the tomatoes, thyme, green (bell) pepper, paprika, chilli powder, chicken stock, sugar and salt. Cook gently until it reduces to a thick paste.

Divide the paste between 4 individual cocotte dishes. Make a small indent in each and crack a whole egg into the centre. Bake in the preheated oven for 12 minutes. Alternatively, put the paste in one ovenproof dish or pan, break in the eggs and cook as above.

Serve hot, sprinkled with chopped parsley and drizzled with olive oil.

NUTRITION FACTS

Tomatoes and peppers are packed with antioxidant beta-carotene and vitamin C, as well as lycopene, which supports prostate health. Eggs supply every nutrient required for healing and repair.

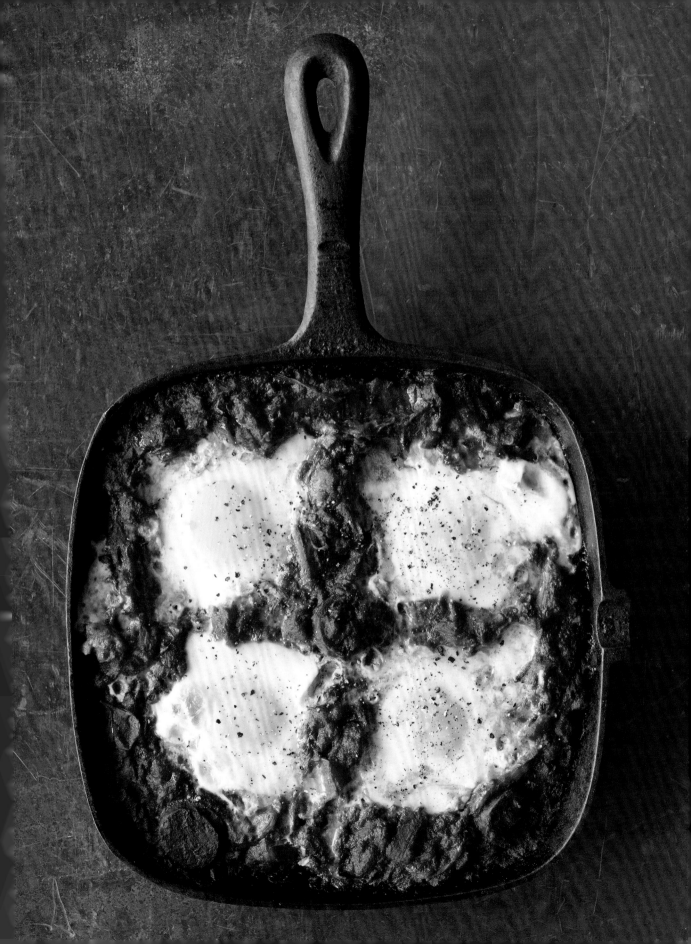

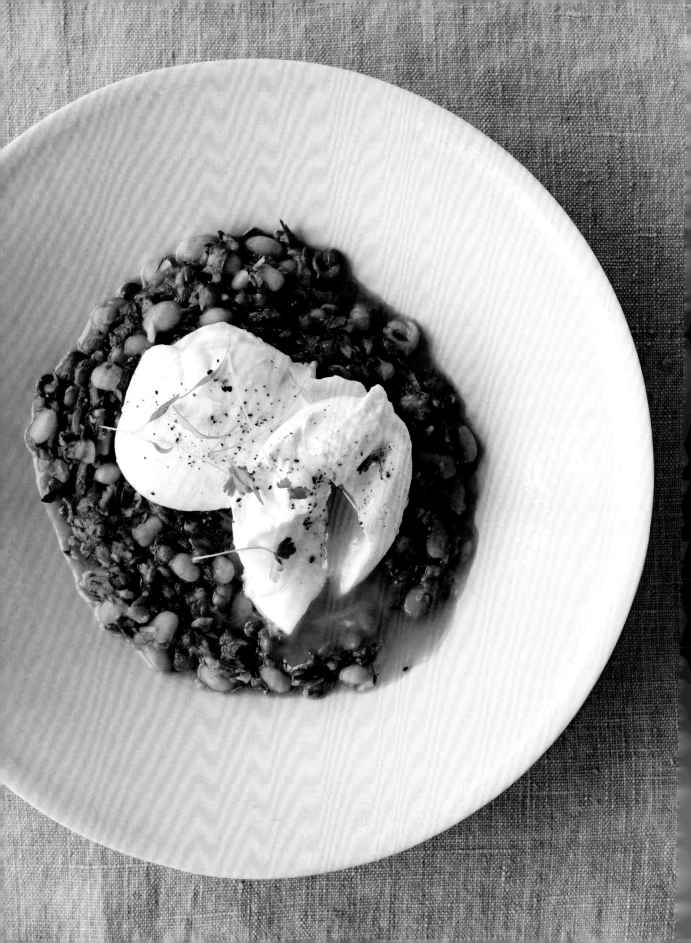

Ⓟ Ful medames with poached eggs

Pulses and lentils are a good source of protein at the beginning of the day. Haricot beans and lentils provide excellent slow-release energy, and soaking overnight to break down the fibre makes them more digestible. Their nutrients are accessed without taxing the digestive system.

Serves 4

20g (¾oz) clarified butter

300g (10oz) onions, thinly sliced

½ tsp ground cumin

1 tsp ground coriander

1 garlic clove, crushed

400ml (14fl oz/1⅔ cups) chicken stock

80g (3oz/generous ⅓ cup) dried haricot beans, soaked in water with lemon juice overnight, then brought to the boil and simmered until soft

40g (1½oz/¼ cup) red lentils, soaked in boiling water with 1 tsp lemon juice

40g (1½oz/¼ cup) Puy lentils, soaked in water with lemon juice overnight, then boiled for 20 minutes

40g (1½oz/¼ cup) green lentils, soaked in water with lemon juice overnight, then boiled for 25 minutes

½ tsp grated unwaxed lemon zest

4 tsp lemon juice

salt and ground black pepper

few sprigs of flat-leaf parsley, chopped

8 organic free-range eggs

dash of vinegar

extra virgin olive oil, for drizzling

In a medium pan, heat the clarified butter and sauté the onions over a medium heat until softened and starting to caramelize, stirring continuously once the onion takes on a little colour.

In the last few minutes, add the cumin, coriander and garlic, and then pour in the chicken stock. Increase the heat and cook rapidly to reduce by half, then add the cooked beans and all the lentils. Continue cooking over a medium heat until most of the stock has been absorbed by the beans and lentils. Add the lemon zest, lemon juice, some salt and pepper and, finally, the chopped parsley.

Poach the eggs in a pan of salted water with a dash of vinegar for 3 minutes. Serve on top of the beans and drizzle with olive oil.

P Coconut, poppy seed, ginger & lime muffins

Coconut flour is the perfect gluten-free choice but you need more fluid than usual. You can eat the muffins as a morning treat whilst adhering to the protein principle of the Plan due to the coconut milk, oil and flour. They can be cooked and then frozen, but are best served fresh with berries.

Makes 12 muffins

80g (3oz) coconut oil, plus extra for greasing the muffin tin

3 organic free-range eggs

200ml (7fl oz/generous ¾ cup) coconut milk

seeds of 1 vanilla pod (bean)

10g (½oz) ground ginger

100ml (3½fl oz/generous ⅓ cup) local runny honey plus extra for the raspberries (optional)

15g (½oz) poppy seeds

grated zest of ½ lime

1 tsp baking powder (baking soda)

40g (1½oz/scant ¼ cup) coconut flour

300g (10oz/2¼ cups) raspberries

fresh coconut and mint leaves, to garnish

Preheat the oven to 180°C, 350°F, Gas mark 4.

In a small saucepan, gently warm the coconut oil – it should be blood temperature rather than too warm. Pour into a large mixing bowl. Add the eggs, coconut milk, vanilla seeds, ginger, honey, poppy seeds and lime zest. Whisk together to make an emulsion.

Mix the baking powder (baking soda) with the coconut flour, then sift into the wet mixture. Using a metal spoon, stir to make a batter.

Divide the mixture between 12 muffin cases or a lightly oiled muffin tin. Bake in the preheated oven for 15 minutes until the muffins are risen and golden brown.

While the muffins are cooking, purée two-thirds of the raspberries. Sweeten to taste, if wished, with a little honey.

Remove the muffins from the oven and set them aside to cool for 10 minutes. Serve warm with the raspberry purée, garnished with the remaining raspberries, fresh coconut and mint.

NUTRITION FACTS

Starting the day with a coconut-rich breakfast helps to balance blood sugar levels and lower cholesterol. This nut-based flour provides abundant Omega-nutrition, which benefits the digestion, waistline, hair and skin.

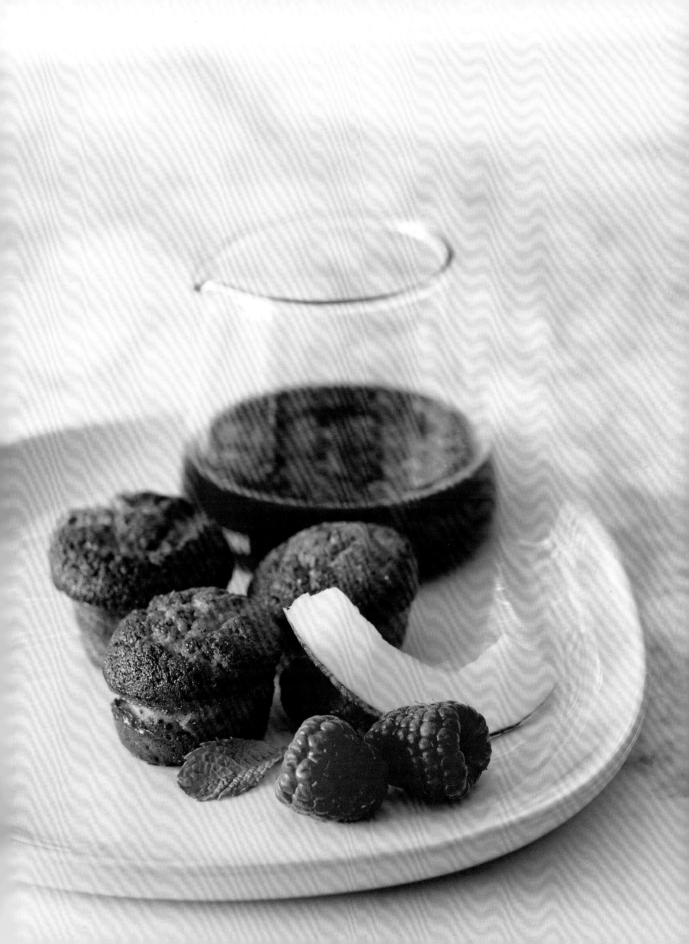

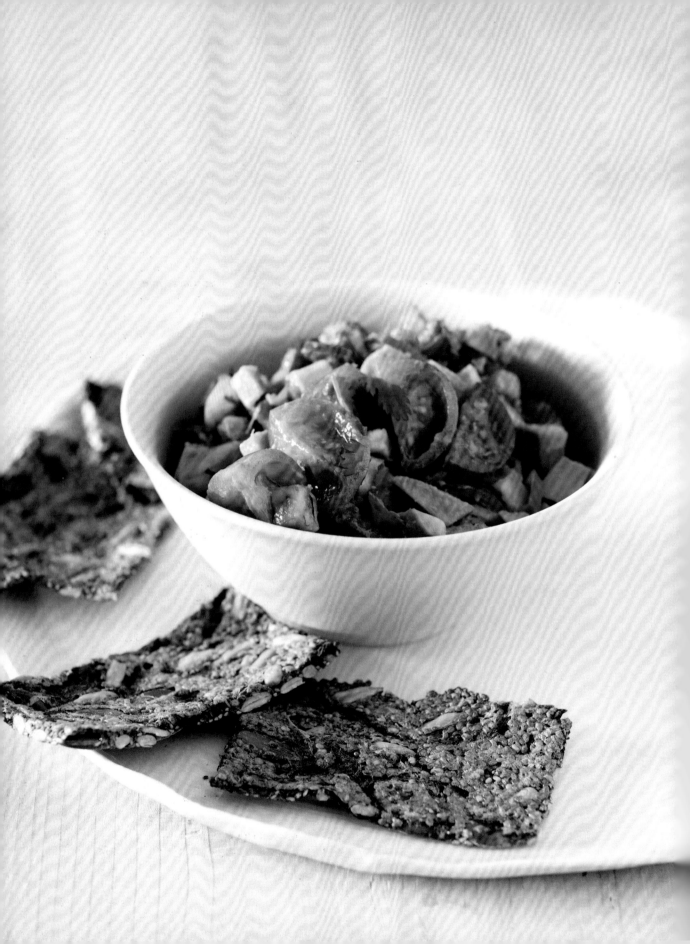

Avocado, chipotle & tomato salsa

Packed with vitamin E, avocados are soothing and simple to digest. Combined with tomatoes, this hot spicy salsa is packed with fresh-tasting antioxidants and can be served with fish, poultry or meat as well as dehydrated crackers (see below) for breakfast. This dish is simple but addictive!

Serves 4

1 tsp dried chipotle chilli
5g (¼oz) fresh root ginger, finely grated
1 tbsp lime juice
½ tsp grated lime zest
20g (¾oz) spring onions (scallions)
pinch of ground cumin
pinch of sea salt
10g (½oz) fresh mint, chopped
10g (½oz) fresh coriander (cilantro), chopped
1 tbsp extra virgin olive oil
150g (5oz) cherry tomatoes, quartered
200g (7oz) avocado, peeled, stoned and diced

Soak the dried chipotle chilli in warm water, then chop it finely.

In a large mixing bowl, mix the ginger, chilli, lime juice and zest, spring onions (scallions), cumin, salt, mint, coriander (cilantro) and olive oil. Add the cherry tomatoes, then mash with a fork to bruise them before mixing in the diced avocado. Store in an airtight container in the fridge for up to 3 days.

Serve with the Beetroot, horseradish & seed crackers (below).

Note: If you like your salsa hot and spicy, add some more chilli.

P Beetroot, horseradish & seed crackers

These crackers may be cooked in a dehydrator or oven. Ideally, you should use a silicone sheet or parchment paper for spreading out the crackers to prevent them sticking.

Makes about 20 crackers

100g (3½oz) chia seeds
50g (2oz/generous ¼ cup) sunflower seeds
50g (2oz/generous ¼ cup) pumpkin seeds
1 garlic clove, grated
40g (1½oz) shallot or onion, finely chopped
80g (3oz) raw beetroot (beet), grated on a large grater
8g (¼oz) horseradish, finely grated
10g (½oz) fresh lemon thyme, finely chopped
large pinch of sea salt
pinch of cayenne pepper

Preheat the oven to 170°C, 325°F, Gas mark 3. Soak the chia seeds in a bowl with 100ml (3½fl oz/generous ⅓ cup) cold water for 10 minutes.

In a large mixing bowl, mix all the ingredients together and then spread them out on a silicone sheet as thinly as possible. Bake in the preheated oven for 12 minutes.

Remove from the oven and carefully slide a palette knife underneath the half-cooked crackers to release them from the sheet onto a chopping board. Cut into long strips, then turn them over and arrange on the sheet. Return to the oven and bake on the other side for a further 10 minutes until the crackers are crisp and cooked.

Cool the crackers on a wire rack. Store in an airtight container for up to 1 week. These crackers are delicious served with your favourite dips and salsas.

Alternative cooking method: Dehydrate the mixture at 130°C, 266°F for 12 hours, turning the crackers after 6 hours.

(P) Asian-style salmon tartar

A mouthwatering dish you can eat any time of the day. The nutritional value of the salmon is preserved by marinating it in the lime juice (citric acid), maximizing the Omega-3. This is fish at its best, with ginger and chilli adding flavour and antioxidant protection for the digestion.

Serves 4

320g (11oz) very fresh salmon fillet, skinned, boned and dark meat just below the skin removed, then cut into 2mm (⅛in) dice

2 spring onions (scallions)

60g (2½oz) cucumber, peeled, deseeded and diced

30g (1¼oz) fresh root ginger, peeled and finely diced

1 fresh red or green chilli, deseeded and finely chopped

4 tsp Thai fish sauce (nam pla)

15g (½oz) fresh coriander (cilantro), finely chopped

juice of 1 lime

To make this dish, you need to have all the ingredients ready prepared in advance.

In a clean large stainless steel bowl, mix together the salmon, spring onions (scallions), cucumber, ginger, chilli, fish sauce and coriander (cilantro). Add the lime juice and stir thoroughly.

Leave for 3 minutes and then, using 2 tablespoons, arrange the tartar on serving plates.

Serve with Cashew, sunflower, chia & wasabi crackers (see below), if liked. Drizzle with a little Chilli, lime, papaya and mint dressing (see page 212).

(P) Cashew, sunflower, chia & wasabi crackers

Prepare these protein- and Omega-nutrition-rich crackers in the oven or a dehydrator. Either way, they are delicious, and cooking at a low temperature prevents the fats in the nuts and seeds from turning rancid. The wasabi paste gives them a kick.

Makes about 20 crackers

150g (5oz/1 cup) cashew nuts, soaked in water for 24 hours

50g (2oz/scant ⅓ cup) sunflower seeds, soaked in water for 24 hours

100g (3½oz) chia seeds, soaked in cold water for 15 minutes

2 tbsp lemon juice

60g (2½oz) shallots

1 garlic clove, crushed

1 green (bell) pepper, stalk removed, deseeded and roughly chopped

10g (½oz) wasabi paste

1 tbsp local runny honey

3 tbsp Tamari

Rinse the cashew nuts and sunflower seeds under running cold water, then drain. Using a jug blender, blitz all the ingredients to form a smooth paste.

Pour the mixture out onto a silicone dehydrator sheet and, using a palette knife, spread it out as thinly as possible. Place in the dehydrator at 130°C, 266°F for 4–5 hours or until you can remove the cracker in one piece.

Turn the mixture out onto a chopping board. Using a large knife, cut it into crackers of the required shape and size before returning them to the dehydrator for a further 3–4 hours to continue drying.

When the crackers are ready, they will be crisp and snap. Keep them in an airtight container and store for up to 4 days.

Note: You can dry these crackers in the bottom of a cool oven at 110°C, 225°F, Gas mark ¼ if you don't have a dehydrator. The key to success is always to use silicone sheets, so the mixture can be removed halfway through drying.

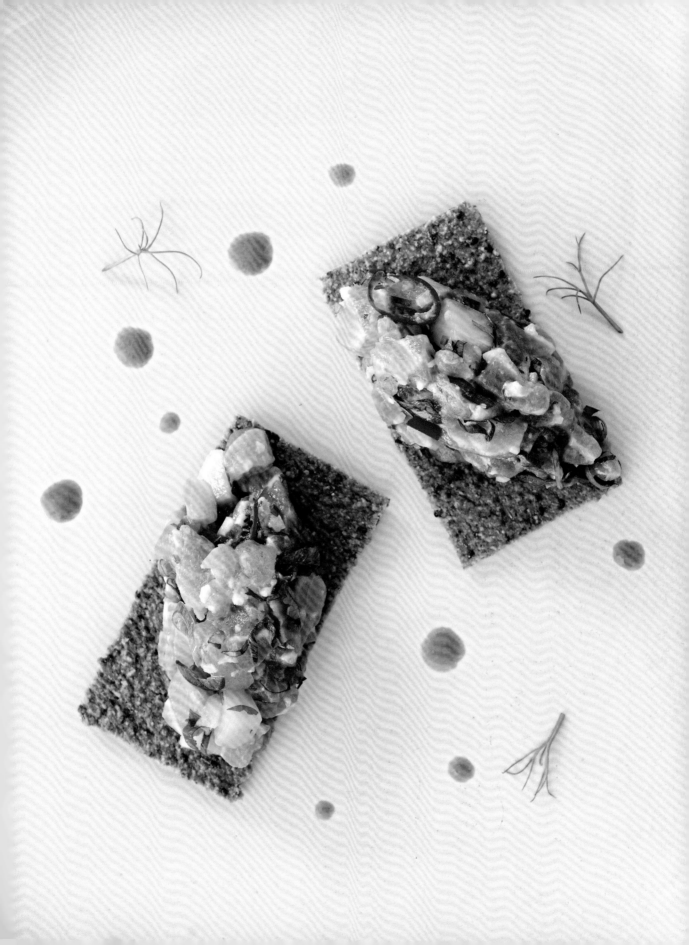

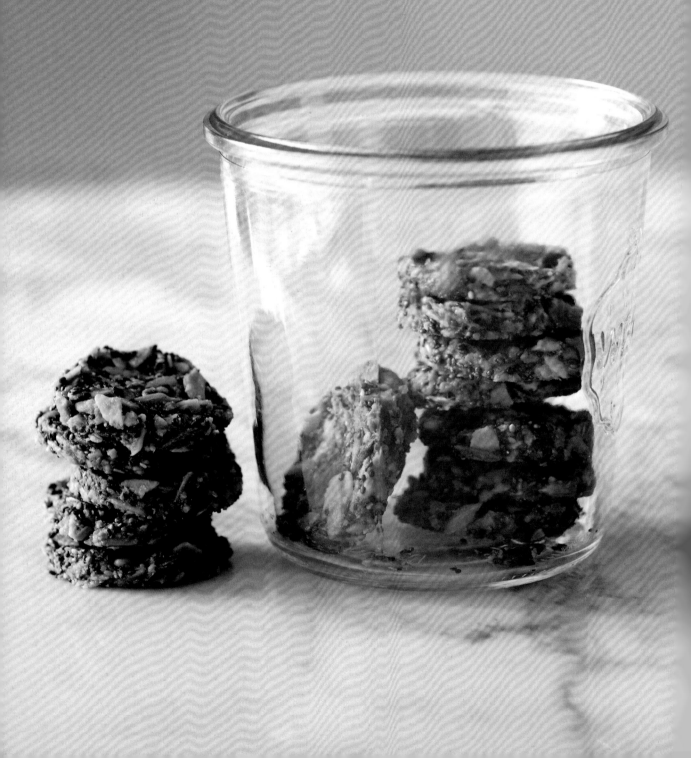

P Chia sweet muesli biscuits

The beauty of using nuts and seeds to make biscuits (cookies) is their texture – crunchy, not crumbly, and sweet, yet satisfying. These little gems can be eaten any time of the day, providing protein and Omega-3 and -6 essential fats. They will satisfy even the most voracious appetite.

Makes 24 biscuits (cookies)

40g (1½oz) coconut oil
2 tbsp maple syrup
10g (½oz) maca powder
50g (2oz/⅓ cup) sunflower seeds
50g (2oz/⅓ cup) pumpkin seeds
20g (¾oz/¼ cup) flaked almonds
40g (1½oz) chia seeds

Melt the coconut oil in a small pan over a low heat. Remove from the heat, add the maple syrup and whisk in the maca powder until everything is well combined.

Stir in the remaining ingredients until thoroughly mixed. Pour the mixture out onto a silicone mat and spread it evenly in a circle.

In a dehydrator, dehydrate for approximately 12 hours at 135°C, 275°F (this may take longer). Check that the mixture is solid but still chewy. Alternatively, put in a cool preheated oven at 110°C, 225°F, Gas mark ¼ for 6 hours, turning the mixture after 3 hours.

Halfway through dehydrating or cooking, remove from the oven and cut into 2.5cm/1in rounds with a metal cutter on a chopping board. Turn the biscuits over and return to the oven.

Using a spatula, remove the mixture from the silicone mat onto a chopping board and cut into 24 pieces.

Keep the biscuits (cookies) in an airtight container at room temperature for up to 1 week.

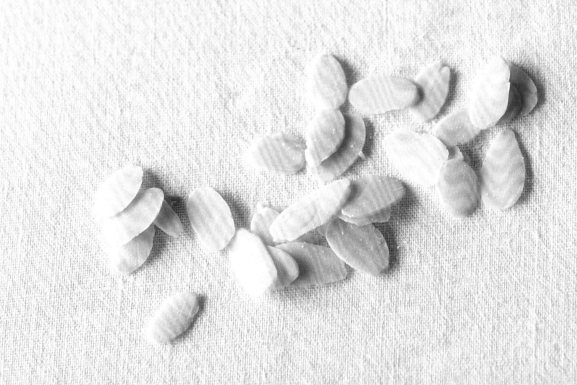

Post-Plan breakfasts

Post-Plan, when all your symptoms have disappeared or have been minimized substantially, breakfast opens up in the grains department, as well as the occasional inclusion of certain cheeses. Buckwheat, millet and oats can be included, and 24-hour fermented yoghurt, full-fat organic cream and natural crème fraîche may also be eaten in moderation.

P+ Savoury goat's cheese flapjack

Filling and full of seeds and goat's cheese, this provides a protein-rich dish or snack that can complete any meal. It may be taken to work with a soup or salad or eaten for breakfast with a smoothie. The chilli and thyme complete the flavouring, making this quite irresistible.

Serves 8

80g (3oz/6 tbsp) unsalted butter

150g (5oz/scant 1 cup) pumpkin seeds

50g (2oz/scant 1/3 cup) sunflower seeds

5g (1/4oz) fresh red chilli, finely chopped

10g (1/2oz) fresh lemon thyme, chopped

1 tsp mixed spice

100g (3½oz) butternut squash, peeled and grated

50g (2oz) local runny honey

4 tsp Tamari

125g (4oz/scant 1¼ cups) rolled oats

125g (4oz) hard goat's cheese, grated

Preheat the oven to 180°C, 350°F, Gas mark 4. Line a round 25cm (10in) flan case with greaseproof paper.

In a thick-bottomed pan, melt the butter. Add the seeds, chilli, thyme and mixed spice and cook gently for about 3 minutes until the seeds just start to pop. Add the butternut squash and cook for 1 minute, then stir in the honey and Tamari.

Remove from the heat and stir in the oats. Mix thoroughly and then add the goat's cheese. Mix again, then spoon into the lined flan case. Level the top, patting it down firmly with a palette knife.

Bake in the preheated oven for 20 minutes until golden brown. Cool in the flan case before removing the flapjack and cutting into slices or wedges. Store in an airtight container in the fridge.

NUTRITION FACTS

Buckwheat contains rutin, which strengthens arterial and micro-capillary walls, as well as iron and calcium for energy and bone health. The fibre in oats regulates blood sugar levels, and the phosphorus repairs cells.

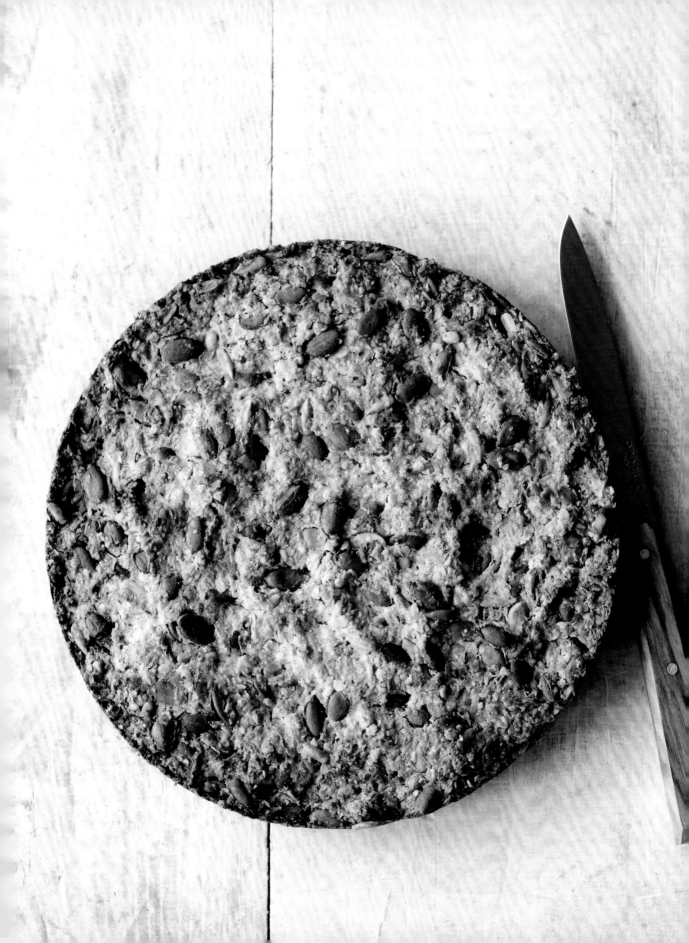

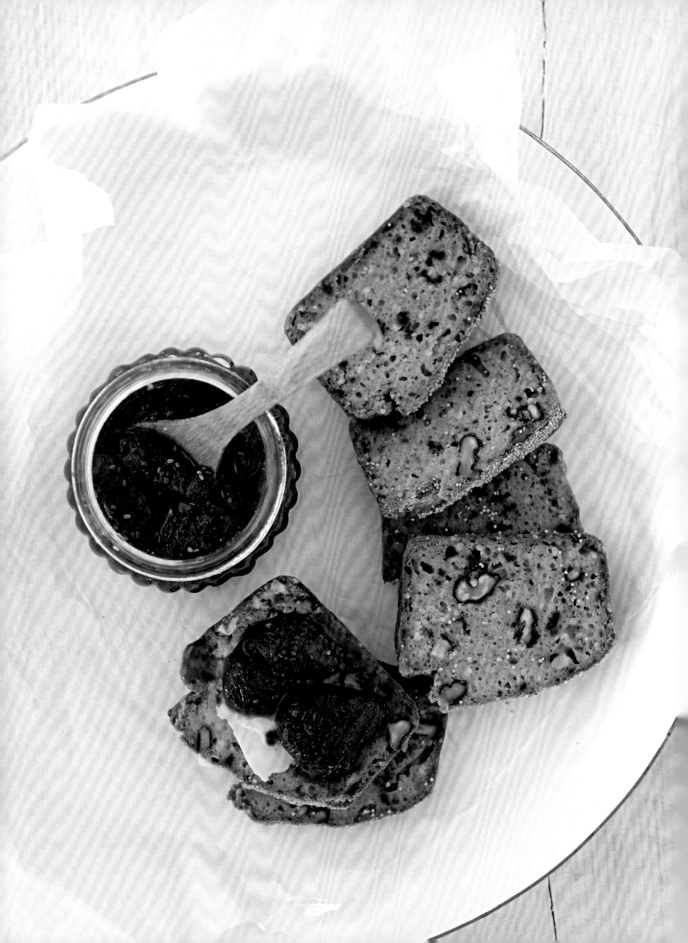

P+ Buckwheat & walnut bread

As non-gluten grains, buckwheat and millet need a combination of arrowroot, egg white and baking powder (soda) to 'bind' the dough, which results in a 'cake' type texture. Adding walnuts and coconut oil makes this a delicious alternative to traditional bread served at breakfast.

Serves 10

200g (7oz/2 cups) buckwheat flour

2 tsp baking powder (baking soda)

40g (1½oz/¼ cup) millet grain

½ tsp arrowroot

pinch of salt

40g (1½oz) coconut oil

300ml (½ pint/1¼ cups) water

1 tbsp lemon juice

½ tsp walnut oil

1 organic free-range medium egg, white only, beaten

40g (1½oz/generous ½ cup) chopped walnuts

Preheat the oven to 180°C, 350°F, Gas mark 4. Line a 450g (1lb) loaf tin with greaseproof paper.

Mix together all the dry ingredients, except the walnuts, in a large bowl. Set aside.

Mix together all the wet ingredients in a separate bowl, then slowly stir it into the bowl of dry ingredients, mixing until you have a wet dough. Add the walnuts and leave to rest for 15 minutes.

Transfer the mixture to the prepared loaf tin and then bake in the preheated oven for 30 minutes until golden brown. Leave the loaf to cool in the tin before turning it out. Store in an airtight container for 3 days. Serve the bread cut into slices with Chia seed, strawberry & orange blossom conserve (see below).

P+ Chia seed, strawberry & orange blossom conserve

This is a wonderful recipe for a fresh short-life, home-made jam, omitting the excessive sugar found in commercial alternatives. Including the orange blossom water and orange zest brings the strawberries alive, whilst the chia adds protein and a thicker, gelatinous texture.

Makes 1 x 450g (1lb) jar

150g (5oz) local runny honey

grated zest of ½ orange

500g (1lb 2oz) strawberries, chopped

10g (½oz) chia seeds

1 tsp orange blossom water

Put the honey, orange zest and strawberries in a thick-bottomed pan and simmer gently for 5 minutes. Add the chia seeds and orange blossom water and remove from the heat.

Ladle the hot strawberry mixture into a clean sterilized jar, then cover and cool before putting the jar into the fridge. Serve chilled.

(P+) Roasted figs with crème fraîche and pistachio mousse

Figs are irresistible in season and taste divine when roasted. They can be prepared the night before and stored in the fridge. The pistachio mousse adds protein to balance the dish, and, when combined with the double cream, provides the CLA (conjugated linoleic acid) that helps with weight loss.

Serves 4

8 fresh figs, quartered

1 tbsp local runny honey

grated zest of ½ lime

½ tsp mixed spice

pistachio powder, to garnish

For the pistachio cream:

50g (2oz) shelled pistachio nuts, ground in a spice blender

50ml (2fl oz/scant ¼ cup) double (heavy) cream

50ml (2fl oz/scant ¼ cup) crème fraîche

few sprigs of fresh mint

juice of 1 lime

2 tbsp local runny honey

Preheat the oven to 180°C, 350°F, Gas mark 4.

Arrange the figs on a non-stick baking sheet. Drizzle with honey and sprinkle the lime zest and mixed spice on top. Roast in the preheated oven for 10 minutes, then remove and allow to cool.

Make the pistachio cream: mix all the ingredients together. Blitz in a jug blender and pass through a fine sieve. Pour into a cream whipper and charge with gas (or beat until stiff).

Arrange the figs (warm or cold) on 4 serving plates and sprinkle with pistachio powder. Fill a small glass with the pistachio mousse.

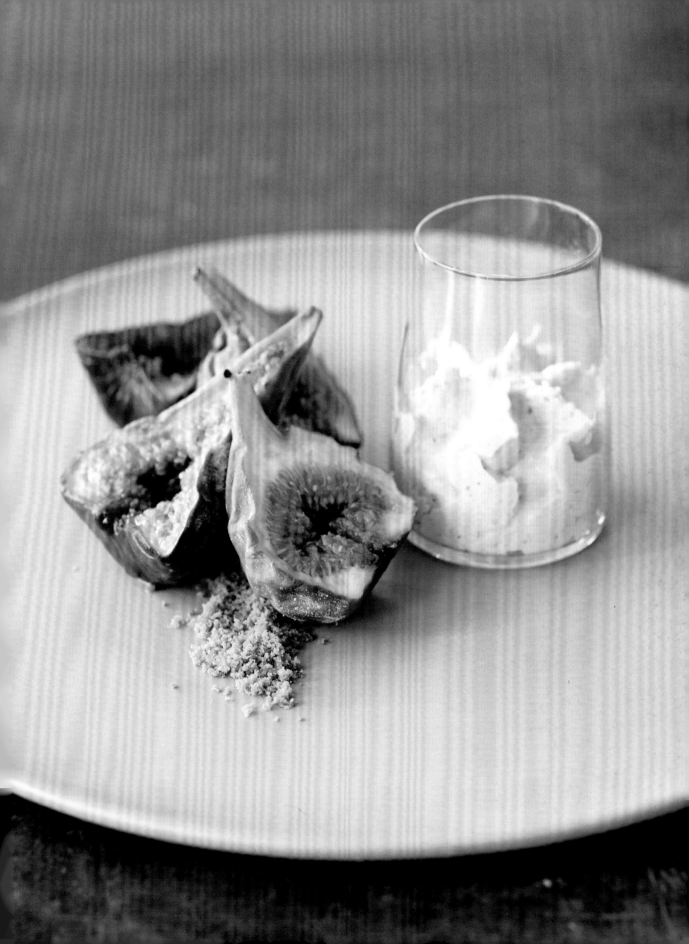

P+ Winter Bircher-style muesli

Soaking the oats and nuts overnight makes them soften and swell, stimulating the enzymes to be activated and making this a more easily-absorbed breakfast for long-lasting energy throughout the morning. Adding natural yoghurt provides probiotics for digestive health.

Serves 4

40g (1½oz/generous ⅓ cup) rolled jumbo oats

20g (¾oz/scant ¼ cup) chopped walnuts

20g (¾oz/scant ¼ cup) hazelnuts

125ml (4fl oz/½ cup) cold water

40g (1½oz/¼ cup) unsulphured dried apricots, cut into 5mm (¼in) slices

60g (2½oz/⅓ cup) prunes, cut into 5mm (¼in) slices

40g (1½oz/¼ cup) dried figs, cut into 5mm (¼in) slices

10g (½oz) fresh root ginger, peeled and finely diced

zest of 1 orange, half removed with peeler and rest finely grated

juice of ½ orange

1 tsp mixed spice

pinch of ground ginger

100g (3½oz) Braeburn apples, skin left on, grated on a large grater

150g (5oz/scant ¾ cup) 24-hour fermented yoghurt (see page 52)

pinch of ground cinnamon

In a bowl, soak the oats and all the nuts in the cold water overnight in the fridge.

Put the apricots, prunes, figs, root ginger, strips of orange zest, orange juice, mixed spice and ground ginger into a small non-aluminium pan. Cover with water and bring to the boil. Reduce the heat and simmer gently for 15–20 minutes until most of the water has been absorbed and the fruit is soft. Allow to cool.

In a mixing bowl, mix the soaked oats and nuts with the grated apple, grated orange zest, yoghurt and cinnamon. Mix thoroughly and spoon into 4 glasses. Top with the cold fruit mixture.

Note: The muesli can be kept in an airtight container in the fridge for a couple of days. If, after several days, the oat mixture becomes stodgy, simply add a little more yoghurt to loosen it.

P+ Summer berry Bircher-style muesli

The cashews and almonds in this version supply abundant magnesium to support heart and nervous system health. The grated pear, whose pectin has an enzymatic action on the oats, renders this muesli very creamy even before the addition of the fermented yoghurt.

Serves 4

40g (1½oz/generous ⅓ cup) jumbo rolled oats

20g (¾oz/scant ¼ cup) chopped cashew nuts

15g (½oz) flaked almonds

125ml (4fl oz/½ cup) cold water

100g (3½oz/⅔ cup) frozen mixed berries

4 tsp local runny honey

100g (3½oz/scant ½ cup) 24-hour fermented yoghurt (see page 52)

seeds of ½ vanilla pod (bean)

100g (3½oz) pears, peeled, cored and grated on a large grater

60g (2½oz/½ cup) strawberries, hulled and sliced

60g (2½oz/½ cup) blackberries

60g (2½oz/½ cup) raspberries

40g (1½oz/generous ¼ cup) blueberries

For the garnish:

8 fresh mint leaves, finely shredded

finely grated zest of ½ lemon

In a bowl, soak the oats and all the nuts in the cold water overnight in the fridge.

Put the frozen berries in a small pan with the honey and bring to a simmer over a low heat. Cook gently for 2 minutes. Pass through a fine sieve while the berries are still hot and then set aside to cool.

In a large mixing bowl, mix the soaked oats and nuts with the yoghurt, vanilla seeds and grated pear. Mix thoroughly and spoon into 4 glasses. Top with the cooled berry mixture and the fresh berries. Serve with shredded mint and finely grated lemon zest.

Note: This muesli can be kept for a couple of days in an airtight container in the fridge. If it's too thick after a couple of days, just add a little more yoghurt to loosen it.

Opposite: Winter Bircher-style muesli (left) and Summer berry Bircher-style muesli

CHEF'S TIP

This muesli may be made well in advance and stored in an airtight container in the fridge to provide you with at least 2–3 days' supply.

P+ Peach & vanilla smoothie with frozen raspberry yoghurt

This is equally suitable for serving as a delicious dessert at a dinner party. The peaches may be cooked and puréed in advance and stored in the fridge, but don't mix with the cream until just before eating. The frozen yoghurt is best eaten on the day it is made as it tends to become icy if kept in the freezer.

Serves 4

4 ripe peaches, halved and stoned

200ml (7fl oz) double (heavy) cream

600g (1lb 5oz) 24-hour fermented yogurt (see page 52)

seeds from 1 vanilla pod (bean)

4 tsp local runny honey

grated zest of ¼ orange

For the frozen raspberry yoghurt:

200g (7oz) frozen raspberries

175g (6oz) 24-hour fermented yoghurt (see page 52), which has been placed in the freezer for 1 hour

50ml (2fl oz/scant ¼ cup) maple syrup

Preheat the oven to 180°C, 350°F, Gas mark 4.

Place the peaches, stoned-side up, on a baking tray lined with parchment paper. Roast in the preheated oven for 20 minutes. Allow to cool.

Make the smoothie: blitz the roasted peaches in a blender until puréed and pass through a fine sieve into a large bowl. In a separate bowl, whisk the cream until it stands in soft peaks. Stir gently into the peach purée. Add the yoghurt, vanilla seeds, honey and orange zest. Mix thoroughly and then divide between 4 glasses. Keep in the fridge until ready to serve.

The frozen raspberry yoghurt can be made in advance if necessary, but it is best made just before serving. Simply blend the frozen raspberries, semi-frozen yogurt and maple syrup together in a jug blender until smooth.

To serve, using an ice cream scoop, scoop out a ball of frozen raspberry yoghurt and place on top of a smoothie. Repeat in the same way with the remaining smoothies and yoghurt.

NUTRITION FACTS

Peaches are packed with valuable bioflavanoids and carotenoids to heal the gut and protect the skin. The fermented yoghurt provides the digestive system with beneficial probiotics to regenerate the intestinal cells.

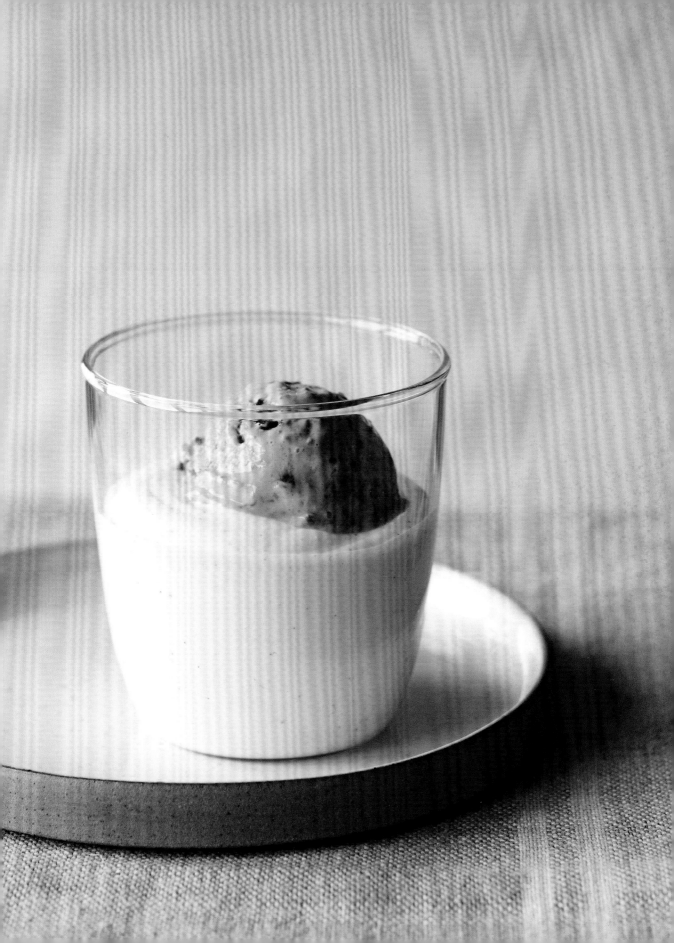

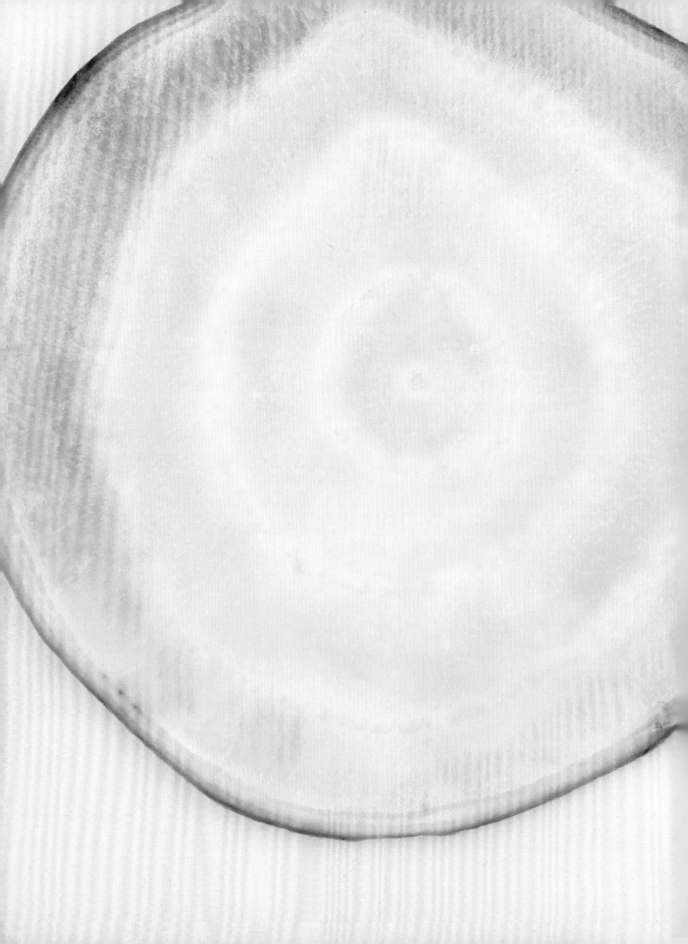

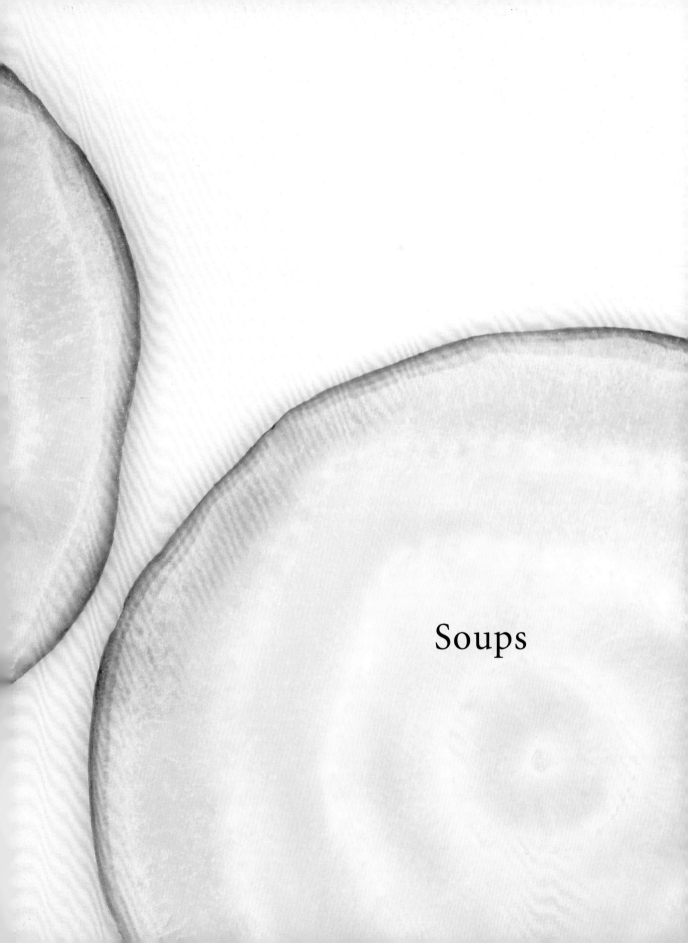

Soups

(P) Moroccan spiced pumpkin soup

Serve this earthy soup hot in winter or chilled in summer. Ras-el-hanout should be a staple in any kitchen – it adds complexity to taste and contains most of the anti-inflammatory spices. Pumpkin has a naturally sweet flavour and also stimulates immunity in the gut.

Serves 4

20g (¾oz) clarified butter

600g (1lb 5oz) pumpkin, peeled, deseeded and cut into 2cm (1in) cubes

80g (3oz) leek, roughly chopped

125g (4oz) carrots, chopped

60g (2½oz) celery, roughly chopped

2 bay leaves

800ml 1⅓ pints/3¼ cups) Chicken Broth (see page 44)

10g (½oz) mint leaves

salt and ground black pepper

4 tsp lemon juice

For the spice mix:

1 tsp grated nutmeg

1 tsp ground cumin

2 pimentos, crushed in a pestle and mortar

½ tsp cayenne pepper

1 tsp paprika

1 cinnamon stick, broken in half

For the garnish:

1 tsp clarified butter

20g (¾oz) pumpkin seeds

½ tsp ras-el-hanout

Preheat the oven to 180°C, 350°F, Gas mark 4.

Melt the butter in a large thick-bottomed pan over a medium heat. Add the pumpkin, leek, carrots and celery, and cook for 10 minutes until golden brown, stirring occasionally.

Add the spice mix and then cook for a couple of minutes, stirring continuously so that the spices don't burn. Add the bay leaves and cover with the chicken stock. Bring to a simmer and cook gently for 20 minutes until the vegetables are tender.

Meanwhile, make the garnish: melt the butter in a pan and stir in the pumpkin seeds and ras-el-hanout. Arrange them on a non-stick baking sheet and bake in the preheated oven for 12 minutes.

Remove the bay leaves and cinnamon sticks and blitz the soup in a blender with the mint until smooth. Season to taste with salt and pepper and lemon juice, then pass through a fine sieve into warmed soup bowls.

Garnish the soup with a sprinkle of the toasted spiced pumpkin seeds and serve immediately.

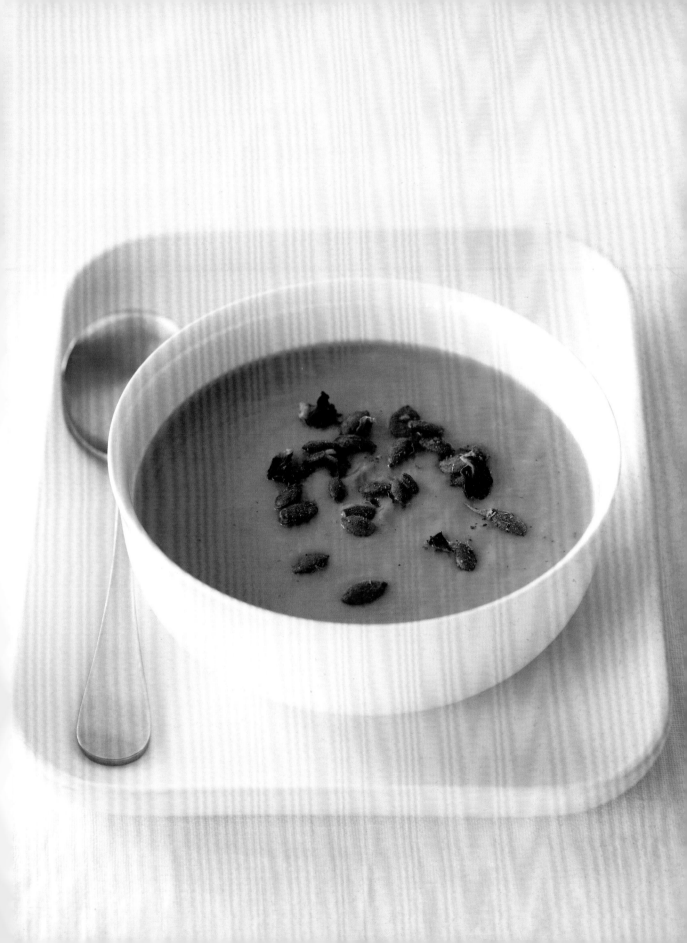

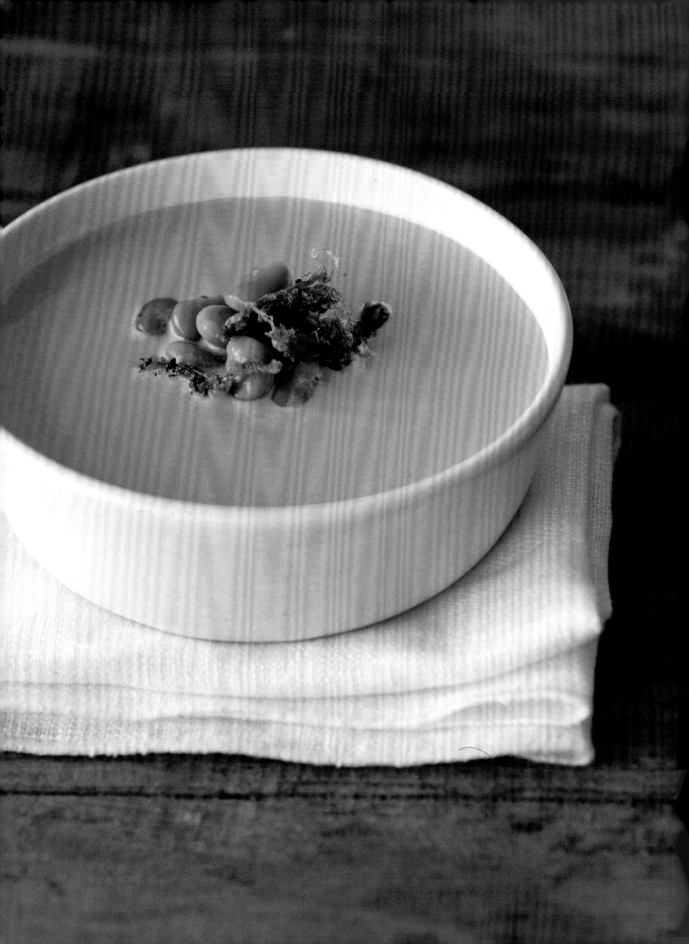

Pea, broad bean & lovage velouté with crispy confit of duck

This is not as complicated as it sounds and you can eat the leftover duck legs as a delicious lunch or supper with some blanched salad or vegetables. The divine velvety soup can be frozen and contains abundant protein from egg yolk, almond milk and broad (fava) beans.

Serves 4

20g (¾oz) butter
100g (3½oz) onion
50g (2oz) celery
50g (2oz) leek
1 garlic clove
few sprigs of thyme, leaves stripped from the stems
2 bay leaves
600ml (1 pint/2½ cups) Chicken Broth (see page 44)
250g (8oz/2 cups) frozen peas
125g (4oz) podded broad (fava) beans
2 organic free-range egg yolks
40ml (1½fl oz/3 tbsp) almond milk
1 tsp chopped lovage
salt and ground black pepper
1 confit of duck leg (see below), to serve

Melt the butter in a small saucepan and then add the onion, celery, leek and garlic. Cook gently until lightly golden. Add the thyme, bay leaves and chicken broth, and bring to the boil. Reduce the heat and add the peas and 100g (3½oz) of the broad (fava) beans (reserve the rest for the garnish). Cook gently for a further 10 minutes.

Blend the egg yolks, almond milk, lovage and salt and pepper in an electric blender. Add the soup, in batches, and blend until smooth. Pass the soup through a fine sieve into a clean pan.

Heat the soup gently over a low heat, taking care that it does not boil as this will cause it to split. Blanch the remaining broad (fava) beans for 1 minute in boiling water, then drain them and remove the skins. Reserve for the garnish.

Remove the skin and bones from the duck leg. Break the flesh apart roughly to shred it. Add the shredded duck to a hot pan and place over a medium heat for 1 minute, stirring continuously to ensure it does not burn. The duck should be crisp.

Ladle the soup into warm bowls, and top with the shredded crispy duck and reserved broad (fava) beans. Serve immediately.

Confit of duck

Duck is far leaner than you might think, as it is a wild bird and packed with flavour. Slow-cooking retains all the taste as well as the nutrients. Cook this in larger batches, if desired.

Makes 4 legs

4 duck legs
100g (3½oz) sea salt
3 star anise
leaves from few sprigs fresh thyme
leaves from few sprigs fresh rosemary,
5g (¼oz) black pepper
4 bay leaves
zest from 1 lemon, cut into thin strips
1 litre (1¾ pints/4 cups) olive oil

Put the duck legs in a bowl and cover with the sea salt, rubbing it in to coat them all over. Cover and leave in the fridge overnight.

The following day, preheat the oven to 170°C, 325°F, Gas mark 3.

Rinse the salt off the duck legs and pat dry with kitchen paper. Place in an ovenproof dish just big enough to lay them flat. Add the star anise, thyme, rosemary, black pepper, bay leaves and lemon zest and cover with oil. Make sure the duck legs are fully covered.

Cover with a sheet of parchment paper and then with aluminum foil. Bake in the oven for 4 hours or until the duck flesh is soft to the touch.

Remove the foil and parchment and leave to rest for 30 minutes before removing the duck legs from the confit mixture.

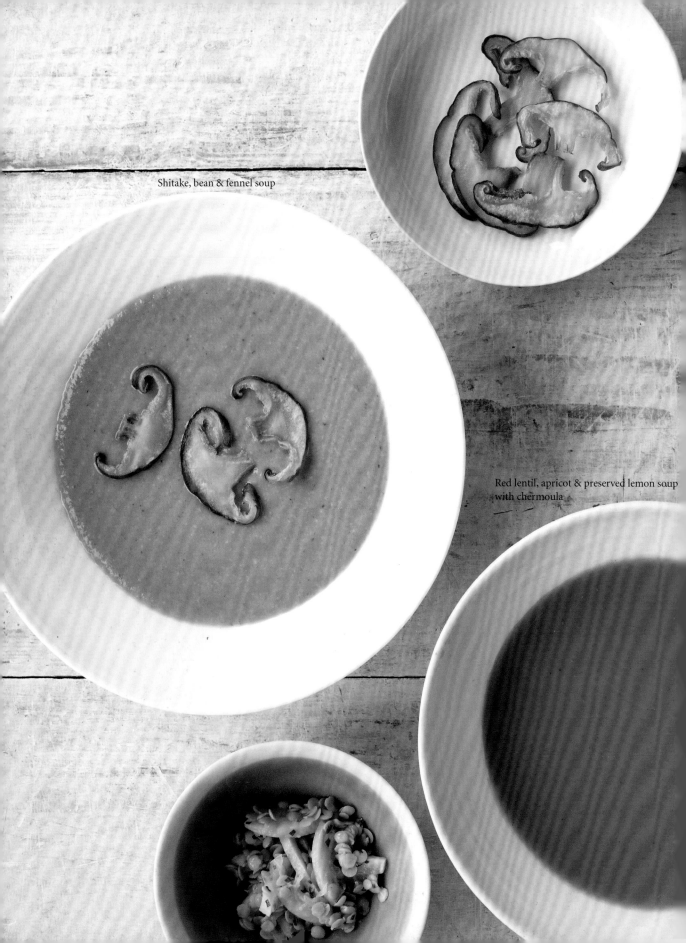

Shitake, bean & fennel soup

Red lentil, apricot & preserved lemon soup
with chermoula

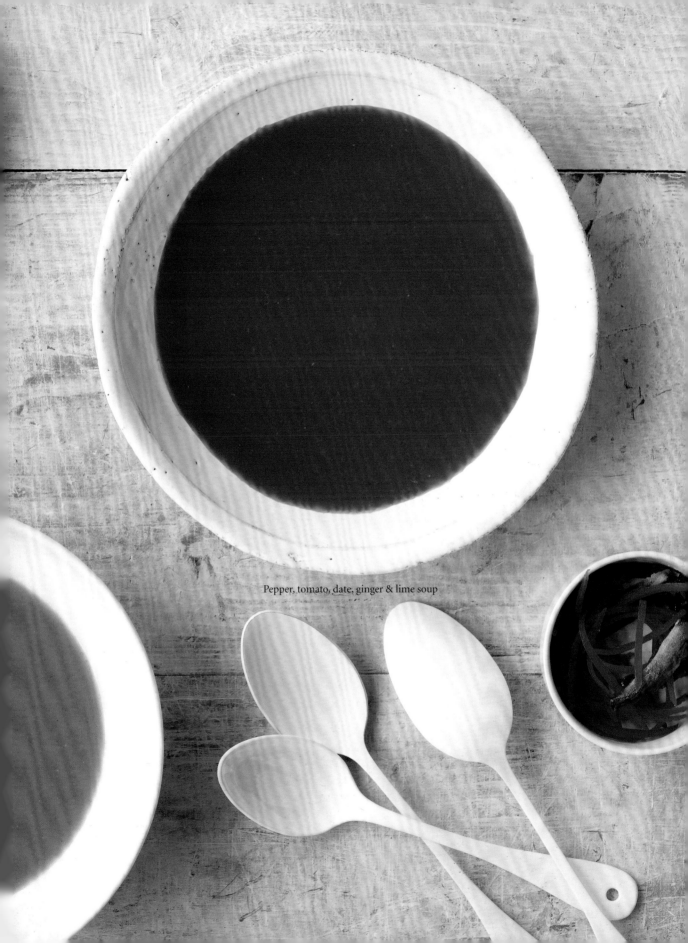

Pepper, tomato, date, ginger & lime soup

ⓟ Shiitake, bean & fennel soup

Using beans to thicken soups creates a smooth and creamy texture. Shiitake mushrooms have been used for thousands of years in Chinese medicine for their immune-stimulating properties, while fennel bulbs and seeds are excellent for cleansing the digestion as well as supporting kidney function.

Serves 4

10g (½oz) coconut oil

200g (7oz) fennel bulb, finely shredded

2 celery sticks, finely shredded

1 onion, finely chopped

100g (3½oz) shiitake mushrooms, sliced

1 garlic clove, crushed

1 tsp fennel seeds

4 thyme sprigs

2 bay leaves

200g (7oz) cooked haricot blanc beans

750ml (1¼ pints/3 cups) Chicken Broth
(see page 44)

salt and ground black pepper

juice of ½ lemon

2 shiitake mushrooms, sliced and
fried in 1 tsp clarified butter

Melt the coconut oil in a thick-bottomed pan. Add the fennel, celery, onion, shiitake mushrooms, garlic and fennel seeds and sweat over a medium heat until they turn a light brown colour.

Stirring continuously, add the thyme, bay leaves and beans and cover with the chicken broth. Simmer for 20 minutes.

Remove the bay leaves and thyme and liquidize the soup, using a stick or jug blender, until smooth. Season with salt and pepper to taste and the lemon juice.

Pass the soup through a fine sieve. Ladle into bowls and serve with the fried shiitake mushrooms.

Illustrated on page 98.

ⓟ Red pepper, tomato, date, ginger & lime soup

Medjool dates impart the distinctive densely sweet flavour of this soup. Tomatoes and red (bell) peppers are both rich in antioxidants, beta-carotene and vitamin C, which, along with the chicken broth, make this an excellent choice for healing and repairing the gut.

Serves 4

2 large red (bell) peppers

200g (7oz) ripe tomatoes, halved

2 tsp coconut oil

100g (3½oz) onion, finely chopped

2 garlic cloves, crushed

20g (¾oz) chopped fresh root ginger

50g (2oz) celery, finely chopped

50g (2oz) carrot, finely chopped

50g (2oz) leek, finely chopped

50g (2oz) Medjool dates, stoned

750ml (1¼ pints/3 cups) Chicken Broth
(see page 44)

juice and grated zest of 1 lime

pinch of sea salt

For the garnish:

20g (¾oz) red (bell) pepper, cut into thin strips

2 Medjool dates, stoned and shredded

Preheat the oven to 180°C, 350°F, Gas mark 4. Place the whole (bell) peppers and halved tomatoes on a baking tray and roast in the preheated oven for 25 minutes until the skins on the peppers have blistered and the tomatoes have caramelized. Peel the peppers and remove the stalks and seeds. Squeeze the seeds out of the tomatoes and discard.

In a thick-bottomed pan, heat the coconut oil and sweat the onion, garlic, ginger, celery, carrot and leek over a medium heat until golden brown. Add the dates, skinned red (bell) peppers and tomatoes and cover with the chicken broth. Simmer gently for 20 minutes. Add the lime juice and zest and salt, and blend until smooth.

Pass the soup through a fine sieve and serve in warmed soup bowls. Garnish with the red (bell) pepper strips and shredded dates.

Illustrated on page 99.

(P) Red lentil, apricot & preserved lemon soup with chermoula

Once you have made this soup, you will appreciate its complexity. Buy or preserve your own lemons, and make more chermoula than needed to use as a dip or base for dressings. The soaked lentils and chicken broth provide enough protein to make this a light evening meal.

Serves 4

10g (½oz) coconut oil

1 onion, finely chopped

3 garlic cloes, crushed

2 carrots, roughly chopped into 5mm (¼in) pieces

1 celery stick, roughly chopped into 5mm (¼in) pieces

¼ tsp cumin seeds

½ tsp coriander seeds

1¼ tsp ground cinnamon

15g (½oz) dried unsulphured apricots

½ tsp ras-el-hanout

1 tsp paprika

150g (5oz) dried red lentils, soaked in boiling water until cold

750ml (1¼ pints/3 cups) Chicken Broth (see page 44)

1 tbsp chopped preserved lemon

For the garnish:

¼ preserved lemon, finely shredded

2 tsp red lentils, soaked in boiling water for 10 minutes

1 tsp chopped parsley

For the chermoula:

½ preserved lemon

3 tbsp chopped coriander (cilantro)

3 tbsp chopped flat-leaf parsley

1 garlic clove, peeled

½ tsp paprika

1 pinch of saffron strands

1 pinch of cumin

½ fresh red chilli, deseeded and finely chopped

4 tbsp extra virgin olive oil

Make the chermoula: put all the ingredients in a food processor and blitz to a smooth paste.

In a thick-bottomed pan, heat the coconut oil and add the onion, garlic, carrots, celery, cumin and coriander seeds, ¼ tsp of the cinnamon and the dried apricots. Sweat over a medium heat, stirring occasionally, until the vegetables are golden brown.

Add the ras-el-hanout, paprika and lentils, and cover with the chicken broth. Simmer for 20 minutes.

Add the preserved lemon and remaining cinnamon. Blend the soup with a stick blender or in an electric blender jug until smooth. Pass the soup through a fine sieve and serve in bowls, garnished with the preserved lemon, lentils and parsley and the chermoula.

Illustrated on pages 98/99.

NUTRITION FACTS

Red lentils are an excellent source of iron, magnesium and vitamin B6 – all vital for energy production.

P Spiced coconut & roasted carrot soup

This is a classic spiced carrot and coconut soup, with a backnote of lime and coriander. The kaffir lime leaves and lemongrass give this dish its distinctive Asian twist, whilst the coconut milk and chicken stock provide the protein portion, as per the Plan's principles.

Serves 4

500g (1lb 2oz) carrots, roughly chopped

5g (¼oz) coriander seeds, crushed

15g (½oz) coconut oil

1 large onion, finely chopped

6g (¼oz) fresh root ginger, finely chopped

1 garlic clove, crushed

2 stalks lemongrass, peeled and chopped

1 small fresh green chilli, deseeded and chopped

1 stick celery, finely chopped

4 kaffir lime leaves

900ml (1½ pints/3⅔ cups) Chicken Broth (see page 44)

200ml (7fl oz/generous ¾ cup) coconut milk

15g (½oz) coriander (cilantro), roughly chopped

salt and ground black pepper

juice of 1 lime

For the garnish:

12 fresh coconut slices

1 small fresh red chilli, deseeded and finely sliced

1 small fresh green chilli, deseeded and finely sliced

Preheat the oven to 180°C, 350°F, Gas mark 4.

Put the carrots and coriander seeds on a baking tray and roast in the preheated oven for 30 minutes until golden brown.

In a thick-bottomed pan, heat the coconut oil and fry the onion with the ginger, garlic, lemongrass, chilli, celery and lime leaves until softened with no colour. Keep the heat low to medium so as not to colour the vegetables and spices – just to bring out their natural sweetness.

Add the roasted carrots and coriander seeds to the pan and then pour over the chicken broth and coconut milk. Bring to a simmer and cook gently for 15 minutes.

Remove the lime leaves and add the coriander (cilantro). Blend until smooth, using a stick blender or jug blender. Season to taste. Add the lime juice and pass through a fine sieve.

Ladle the soup into bowls and serve garnished with the sliced coconut and red and green chillies.

NUTRITION FACTS

Coriander seeds contain palmitic and oleic acids, which are also found in olive oil and palm oil and are highly anti-inflammatory and antioxidant.

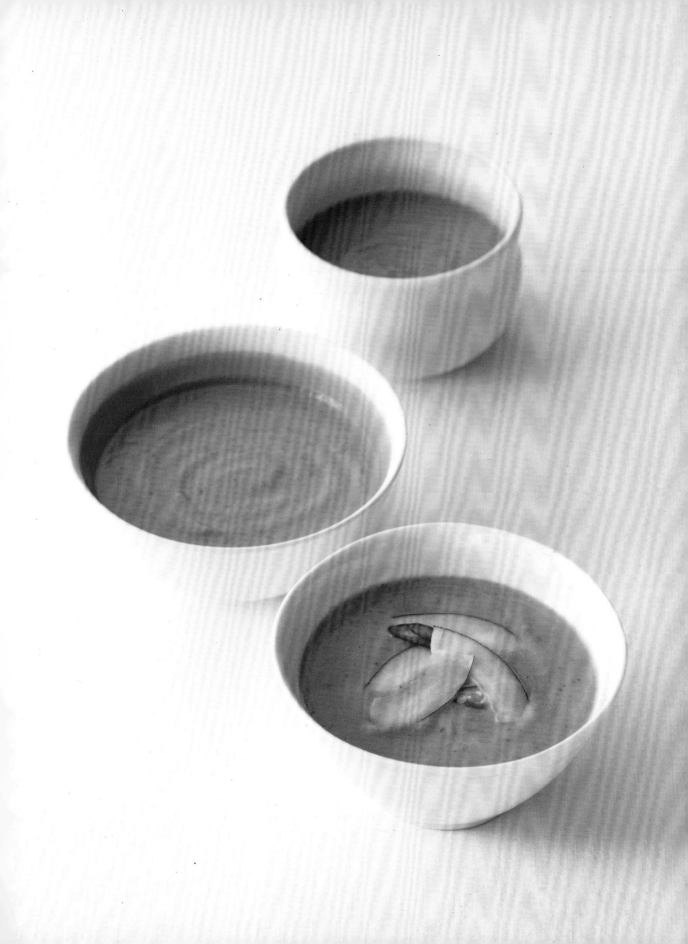

P Roasted beetroot & celeriac soup

This recipe perfectly balances these two root vegetables, so they don't overpower each other, with a smattering of caraway to complement the beetroot (beets). Rich in beta-carotene and vitamin C, beetroot (beets) supports the digestion's liver function, helping to clear toxins.

Serves 4

400g (14oz) beetroot (beets), peeled and cut into 2cm (1in) pieces

400g (14oz) celeriac, peeled and cut into 2cm (1in) pieces

10g (½oz) coconut oil

2 large onions, finely chopped

3 garlic cloves, crushed

2 celery sticks, finely chopped

50g (2oz) leek, finely chopped

½ tsp caraway seeds

800ml (1 pint 7fl oz/3¼ cups) Chicken Broth (see page 44)

2 bay leaves

6 sprigs of thyme

2 tbsp cider vinegar

salt and ground black pepper

Preheat the oven to 180°C, 350°F, Gas mark 4.

Place the beetroot (beets) and celeriac on a non-stick baking tray and roast for 30 minutes until golden brown.

Heat the coconut oil in a thick-bottomed pan, and sweat the onions, garlic, celery, leek and caraway seeds over a medium heat, stirring occasionally with a wooden spoon, until golden brown. Add the roasted beetroot (beets) and celeriac and cover with the chicken broth. Add the bay leaves and thyme.

Simmer gently for 15 minutes. Remove the bay leaves and thyme, and add the cider vinegar. Blend until smooth with a hand blender or jug blender. Pass the soup through a fine sieve and season to taste with salt and pepper.

Serve the hot soup garnished, if wished, with celery leaves and a little Beetroot & caraway dressing (see below).

P Beetroot & caraway dressing

This potent little dressing may also be used as a separate dressing, in its own right, with the blanched salad recipes. Make it in advance, if wished, and store in the fridge for several days.

Serves 4

5g (¼oz) caraway seeds

50g (2oz) beetroot (beet), grated

50ml (2fl oz/scant ¼ cup) Chicken Broth (see page 44)

4 tsp olive oil

4 tsp cider vinegar

salt and cayenne pepper

In a small pan, toast the caraway seeds for a couple of minutes, then add the grated beetroot (beet) and chicken broth. Cook gently over a low heat for 10 minutes until the beetroot is cooked.

Using a hand blender, blend with the olive oil and cider vinegar, and then pass through a fine sieve. Season lightly with salt and cayenne. This will give you a very intensely flavoured dressing.

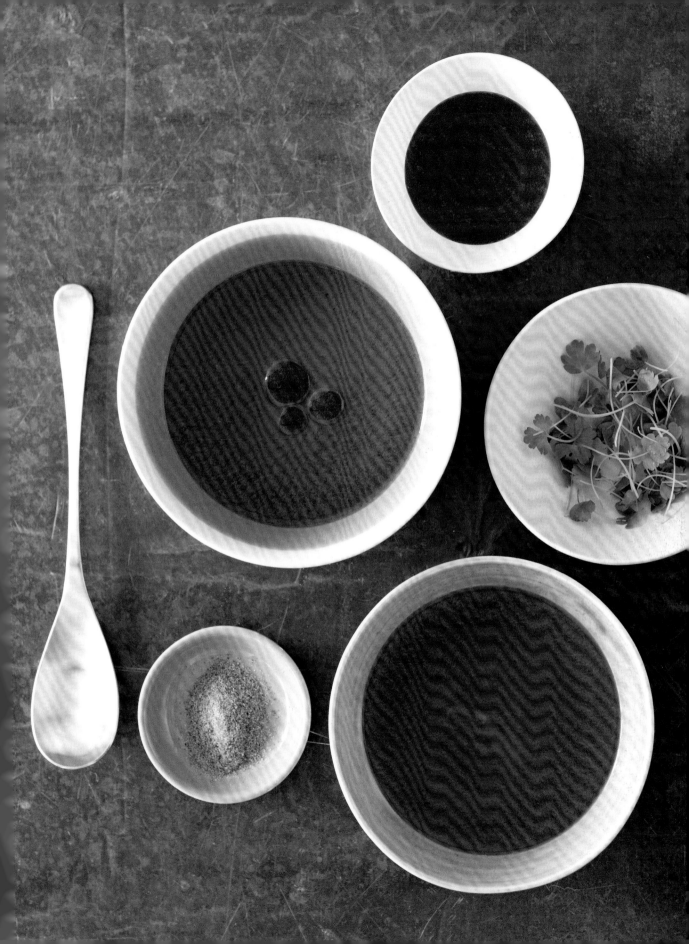

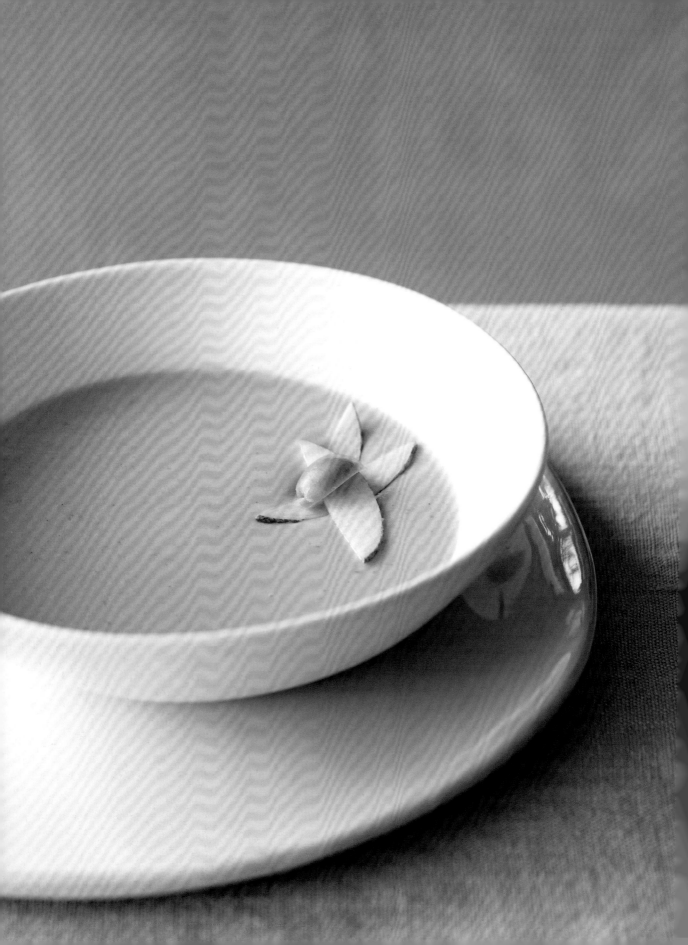

(P) Smokey aubergine soup with peach & green olives

This soup is based on a classic Baba Ganoush, with the unusual addition of sweet peach and salty olives. The smokey taste that comes from cooking the aubergine (eggplant) in its skin has a natural balancing sweetness. Tahini, which is made from sesame seeds, provides the protein.

Serves 4

2 aubergines (eggplants)
10g (½oz) coconut oil
1 onion, sliced
2 garlic cloves, crushed
1 leek, white only, chopped
1 celery stick, chopped
½ tsp ground cumin
600ml (1 pint/2½ cups) Chicken Broth (see page 44)
1 tbsp tahini
pinch of celery salt
10g (½oz) flat-leaf parsley
juice of ½ lemon
ground black pepper

For the garnish:

1 ripe peach, stoned and cut into 1cm (½in) chunks
8 green olives, pitted and sliced

Heat a large frying pan over a high heat. Place the whole aubergines (eggplants) in the dry pan and let them blister all over, turning them occasionally. The skin will burn and the flesh will cook while developing a delicious smoky flavour. This will take 20–30 minutes.

The aubergines (eggplants) are cooked if the flesh is soft when you press it and all the skin is blackened and charred. Allow to cool before using a spoon to remove the cooked flesh. Discard the skin.

In a thick-bottomed pan, heat the coconut oil and sweat the onion, garlic, leek, celery and cumin for about 10 minutes, until soft but not coloured. Stir frequently while the vegetables are sweating.

Add the cooked aubergine (eggplant) flesh and cover with the chicken broth. Bring to a simmer and cook for 15 minutes.

Remove from the heat, and add the tahini, celery salt, parsley, lemon juice and some black pepper. Blend until smooth with a stick blender or jug blender.

Pass the soup through a sieve into soup bowls and garnish with the peach chunks and sliced green olives as shown opposite. This soup can be served hot or cold.

NUTRITION FACTS
Cumin has excellent anti-inflammatory properties and is a brilliant spice for healing the digestive tract.

Ⓟ Chilled broccoli, avocado, almond & mint soup

This beautiful velvety soup is packed with vegetables, and brought to tangy freshness with the mint, lime and avocado. Mint is soothing to the gut, while cardamoms are a rich source of calcium, magnesium and iron, to support growth and repair, and healthy heart function.

Serves 4

10g (½oz) coconut oil

1 small fresh green chilli, deseeded and finely chopped

1 onion, finely chopped

2 celery sticks, chopped

1 leek, white only, finely shredded

1 garlic clove, crushed

8 green cardamom pods

2 bay leaves

75g (3oz/½ cup) almonds, soaked in cold water for 12 hours

700ml (1 pint 3½fl oz/2¾ cups) boiling Chicken Broth (see page 44)

150g (5oz) broccoli florets, very finely shredded (stalks discarded)

1 ripe avocado, about 180g (6oz), peeled, stoned and roughly chopped

juice of 1 lime

pinch of sea salt

15g (½oz) mint leaves

To garnish:

½ avocado, stoned, peeled and diced

8 whole almonds, grated

Heat a thick-bottomed large pan and melt the coconut oil. Add the chilli, onion, celery, leek, garlic and cardamoms and sweat slowly over a low heat without colouring. When everything is soft, add the bay leaves, almonds and chicken broth and bring to the boil.

Add the shredded broccoli and cook for 4 minutes. It is important that you use just the flowering part of the broccoli, not any tough stalks, as these will take too long to cook and you will lose the lovely green vibrancy of the soup.

Remove from the heat and take out the bay leaves before adding the avocado, lime juice and salt. Blend with a stick blender or jug blender until smooth, and then blend the mint into the soup. Pass through a fine sieve into a bowl.

Chill the soup in the fridge before serving. Garnish with diced avocado and grated whole almonds.

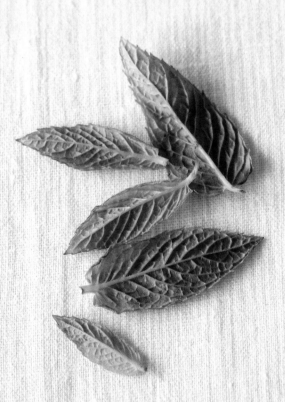

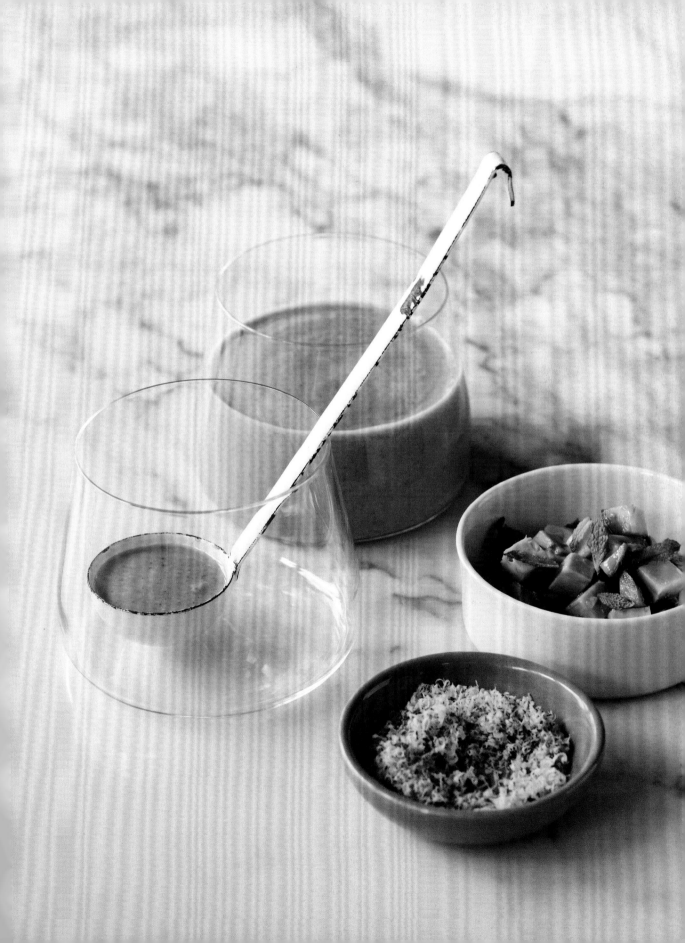

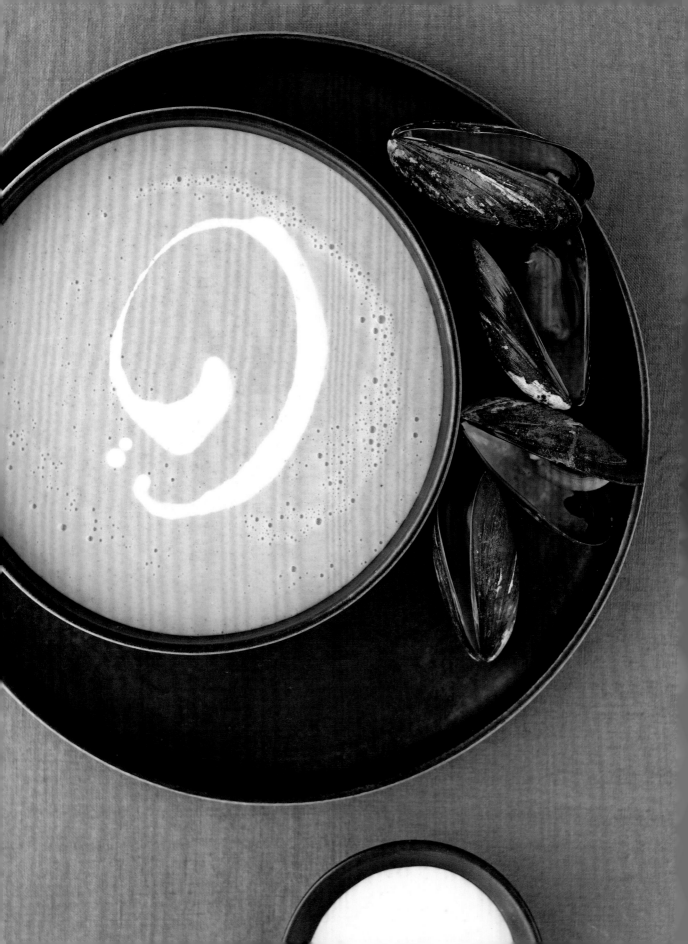

Post-Plan soups

Now that you've completed the Plan, you can start adding chickpeas, borlotti beans and some dairy produce to soups to make them richer in flavour and more substantial. If you've opted not to reintroduce cow's dairy produce, consider goat's and sheep's milk and cheeses as a possible substitute – they tend to be more digestible than the cow's alternatives.

P+ Fennel & mussel velouté with saffron crème fraîche

Serve this divine soup for a dinner party, and your guests will certainly come back for more! Select only the freshest live mussels, and make sure you clean them well before cooking. The fennel, celery and leek all aid digestion, as well as providing balance for the shellfish.

Serves 4

2kg (4lb 7oz) live mussels, cleaned, scrubbed and beards removed

40ml (1½fl oz/3 tbsp) white wine

10g (½oz) clarified butter

500g (1lb 2oz) fennel bulb, choppped,

1 onion, chopped

3 celery sticks, chopped

1 leek, chopped

1 litre (1¾ pints/4 cups) fish stock

2 star anise

1 organic free-range egg yolk

2 tbsp double (heavy) cream

For the saffron crème fraîche:

pinch of saffron strands soaked in 1 tsp water

80ml (3fl oz/scant ⅓ cup) crème fraîche

1 tsp toasted fennel seeds, ground into a powder in a pestle and mortar and passed through a fine sieve

pinch of sea salt

Place a large saucepan over a high heat. Add the mussels and wine, then cover the pan with the lid and steam for 3–4 minutes until the mussels open. Remove from the heat and transfer the mussels to a bowl (reserving the cooking liquor).

Throw away any unopened mussels. Remove the mussel meat from the opened shells, removing any 'beards'. Set aside 12 mussels in their shells for the garnish.

To make the soup, heat a large pan over a medium heat. Melt the butter and sauté the fennel, onion, celery and leek until soft but not coloured. Add the fish stock, the mussel cooking liquor and star anise. Bring to a simmer and cook gently for 20 minutes.

To make the saffron crème fraîche, mix all the ingredients together in a small bowl and reserve for the garnish.

To finish the soup, remove the star anise and blitz in a blender – or use a hand blender – until smooth and pass through a fine sieve into a clean saucepan. Heat through gently without boiling.

Whisk the egg yolk and cream together. Remove the soup from the heat and whisk in the creamy egg mixture. Add the mussel meat and leave for 2 minutes before ladling into soup bowls.

Serve the soup with a swirl of the saffron crème fraîche.

P+ Tomato & bean soup with goat's cheese panatellas & pesto

This great meal-in-a-bowl soup can be eaten without the goat's cheese and basil panatellas if you want a simple supper, but they do complete the dish beautifully if you are entertaining. The pesto is essential for the Italian approach and can be made in larger batches and used with other recipes.

Serves 4

150g (5oz) borlotti beans, soaked overnight in water with lemon juice

knob of clarified butter

1 onion, finely chopped

2 celery sticks, roughly chopped

1 small leek, roughly chopped

1 carrot, roughly chopped

1 garlic clove, sliced

few oregano sprigs, leaves stripped from stalks

pinch of salt

300ml (½ pint/1¼ cups) strained passata

300g (10oz/1½ cups) canned tomatoes

50g (2oz) sun-dried tomatoes, soaked overnight

750ml (1¼ pints/3 cups) Chicken Broth (see page 44)

For the goat's cheese & basil panatellas:

80g (3oz) semi-soft goat's cheese

4 slices Parma ham

4 large basil leaves

1 tsp clarified butter

For the pesto:

50g (2oz) basil leaves

1 small garlic clove, peeled

80ml (3fl oz/scant ⅓ cup) extra virgin olive oil

30g (1oz/scant ¼ cup)) toasted pine nuts (pignoli)

salt and ground black pepper

30g (1oz/¼ cup) grated Parmesan

For the vegetable garnish:

1 courgette (zucchini), cut into 1cm (½in) dice

1 carrot, cut into 1cm (½in) dice

2 celery sticks, cut into 1cm (½in) dice

small piece of clarified butter

Drain the soaked borlotti beans and cook in a pan of boiling unsalted water for 30 minutes. Drain well and set aside.

Make the pesto (in advance, if wished) by pounding all the ingredients in a pestle and mortar until smooth. Cover and leave in a cool place.

To make the soup, melt the butter in a large saucepan and fry the onion, celery, leek and carrot until golden brown. Add the garlic, oregano and salt. Cook for a further 2 minutes, then add all the remaining ingredients. Simmer gently for 15 minutes over a low heat. Remove from the heat and add half the cooked beans, reserving the rest for the garnish, and blitz in a jug blender.

To make the panatellas, split the cheese into 4 equal chunks. Using your hands, roll them into 5cm (2in) long cigar shapes. Lay the Parma ham on a chopping board and place a basil leaf on each slice together with a 'cigar' of goat's cheese. Roll up in the ham and sauté in the butter just before serving.

Just before serving, sauté the vegetable garnish and reserved borlotti beans in a pan over a medium heat until light brown.

Serve the soup warm over the vegetable garnish, with a good dollop of pesto and the panatellas on the side.

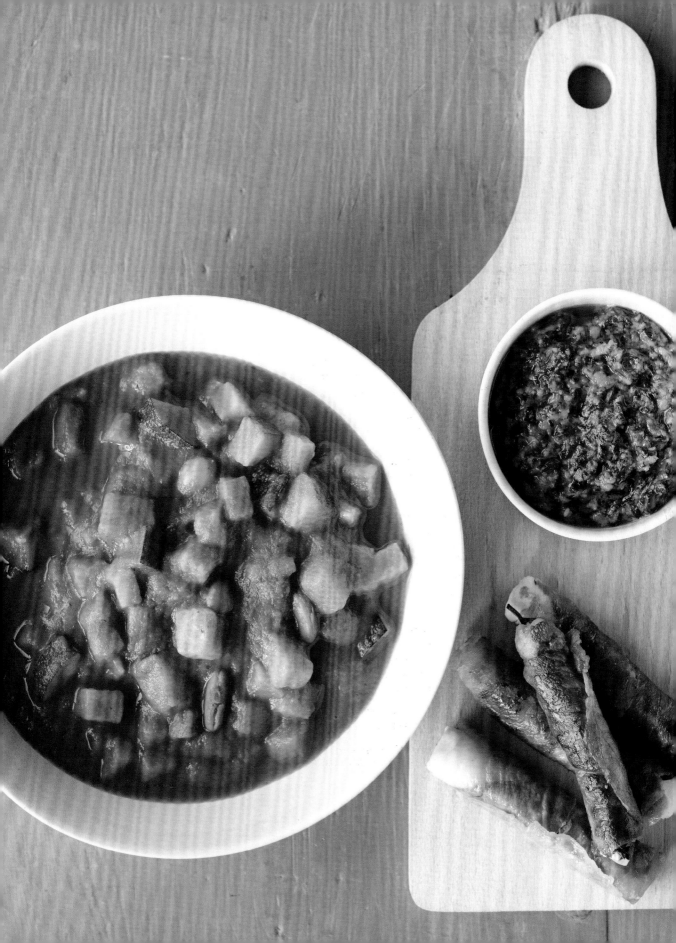

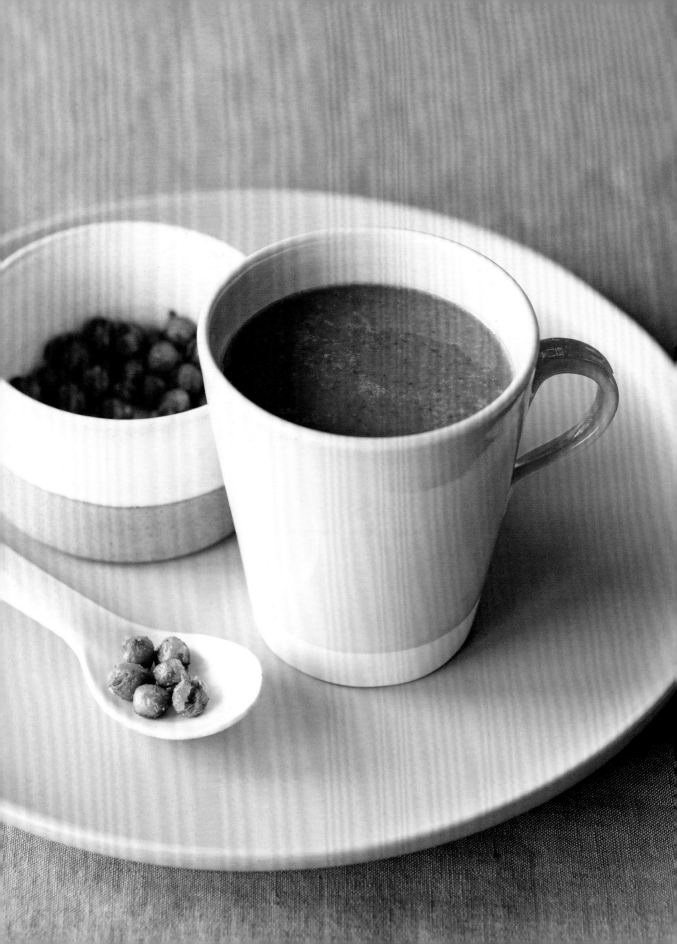

P+ Chickpea, wild garlic & spinach soup

The flavour of fresh wild garlic is worth foraging for, and you will be surprised just how close by some might be growing to you. This is a thicker and richer take on a conventional spinach soup, with the honey adding an unexpected sweet kick.

Serves 4

10g (½oz) clarified butter

100g (3½oz) shallots, diced

2 celery sticks, diced

1 carrot, diced

1 tsp coriander seeds

2 bay leaves

1 small fresh green chilli, deseeded and roughly chopped

300g (10oz/1½ cups) cooked chickpeas

1.2 litres (2 pints/5 cups) Chicken Broth (see page 44)

150g (5oz) baby spinach leaves

30g (1¼oz) wild garlic

4 tsp local runny honey

4 tsp lime juice

pinch of salt

For the garnish:

10g (½oz) clarified butter

100g (3½oz/½ cup) cooked chickpeas

1 tsp curry powder

Preheat the oven to 180°C, 350°F, Gas mark 4.

Heat the clarified butter in a thick-based pan over a medium heat and sauté the shallots, celery, carrot, coriander seeds, bay leaves and chilli until golden brown.

Add the chickpeas and chicken broth and cook for 20 minutes over a low heat. Add the spinach, wild garlic, honey and lime juice, and blend until smooth in a jug blender. Season to taste and pass the soup through a fine sieve.

Meanwhile, make the garnish. Heat the butter in a small pan over a medium heat, then add the chickpeas and curry powder. Cook for 2 minutes, then transfer to a non-stick baking sheet and cook in the preheated oven for 15–20 minutes until the chickpeas are crisp.

Serve the hot soup topped with the garnish of crispy chickpeas.

NUTRITION FACTS

Soaking the chickpeas for 24 hours to remove the phytates is a must for any recipe that includes them, as this makes them far more digestible. Wild garlic is far more potent than farmed alternatives.

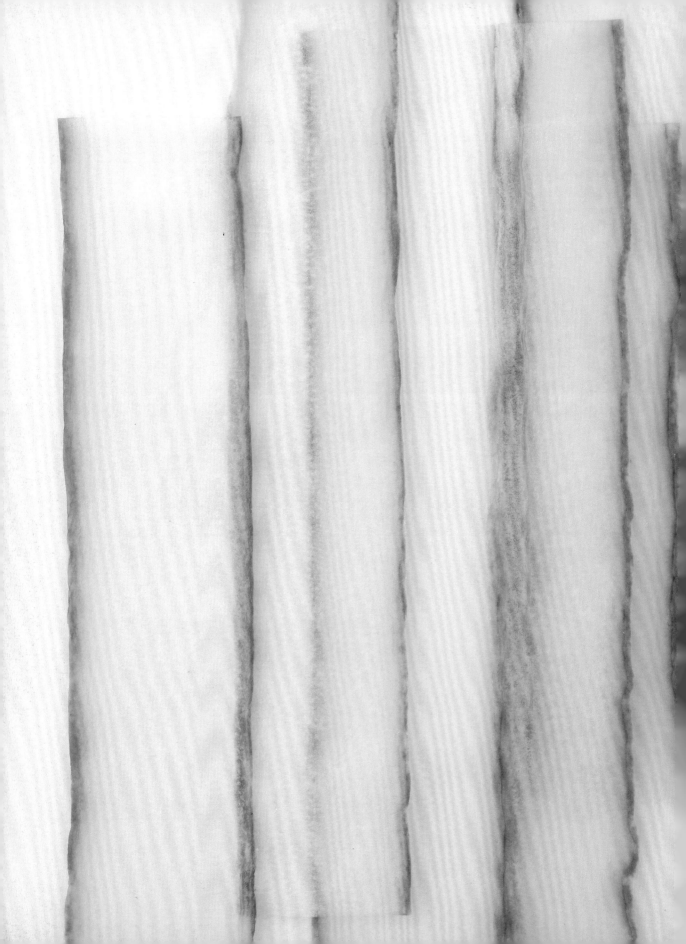

Everyday meals

ⓟ Beef carpaccio with pepper, chilli, ginger & sesame dressing

There is no more pure and unadulterated a dish than one that is raw – good-quality grass-fed beef contains the highest amount of protein, and eating it with a nutritious dressing makes this a balanced meal in itself. With a handful of greens and a blanched salad it's unbeatable.

Serves 8–10

1 tsp coriander seeds, toasted

1 tsp fennel seeds, toasted

½ tsp black peppercorns

pinch of sea salt

500g (1lb 2oz) beef fillet (middle cut), fat and sinews removed

For the dressing:

1 red (bell) pepper

4 tsp extra virgin olive oil

1 tbsp sesame oil

1cm (½in) fresh root ginger, peeled

1 garlic clove, peeled

1 tbsp Tamari

2 tbsp cider vinegar

1 fresh red chilli, deseeded

juice of 1 orange

1 tsp grated orange zest

For the salad garnish:

few sprigs of baby coriander (cilantro)

a little Shiso cress

a few rock chives

toasted black and white sesame seeds for sprinkling

Grind the coriander and fennel seeds with the black peppercorns in a spice grinder or pestle and mortar and then add the salt.

Place a sheet of cling film (plastic wrap) on a clean work surface. Scatter with half of the spice mixture and place the beef fillet on top. Sprinkle the rest of the spice mixture over the beef. Work it into the meat by rolling the fillet back and forth, until it is evenly coated. Roll up tightly in the cling film (plastic wrap) to make a cylinder shape, twisting the ends securely to seal them. Place in the freezer for about 1½ hours until semi-frozen.

Preheat the oven to 200°C, 400°F, Gas mark 6.

Make the dressing: place the red (bell) pepper on a non-stick baking tray and roast for 25 minutes or until the skin blisters and the pepper is soft. Set aside to cool a little, then peel away the skin and remove the ribs and seeds. Using a hand or jug blender, blitz the red (bell) pepper flesh wth all the other dressing ingredients until smooth. Pass the dressing through a fine sieve.

To serve, slice the beef very thinly and arrange on a large serving platter. Mix the salad garnish ingredients together and pile in the middle of the plate. Drizzle with the dressing and sprinkle with toasted sesame seeds.

CHEF'S TIP
To slice the beef fillet ready to serve, always use a very sharp knife. It is worth investing in a good one.

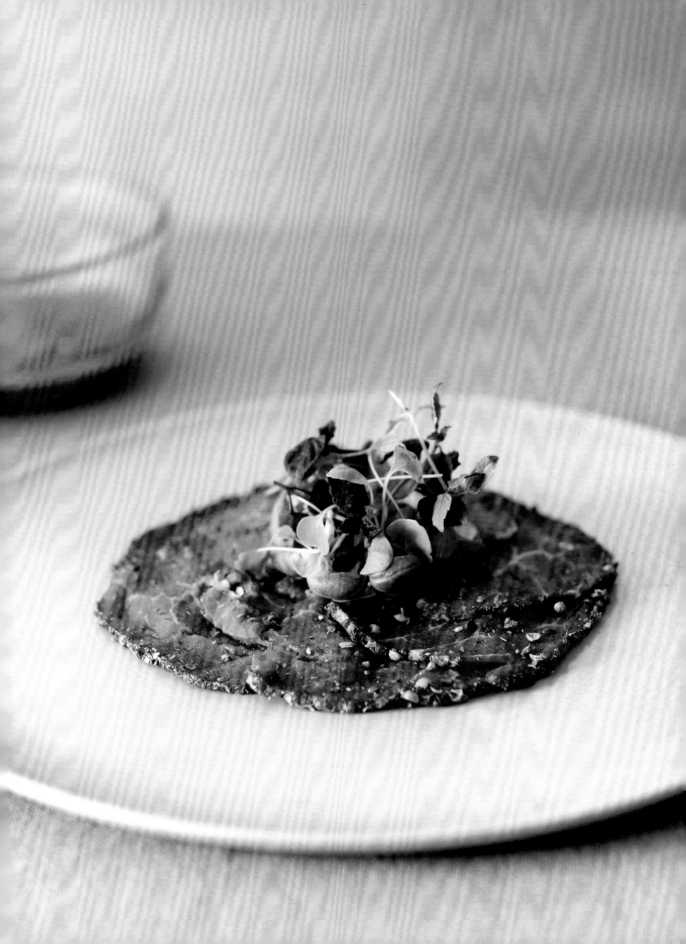

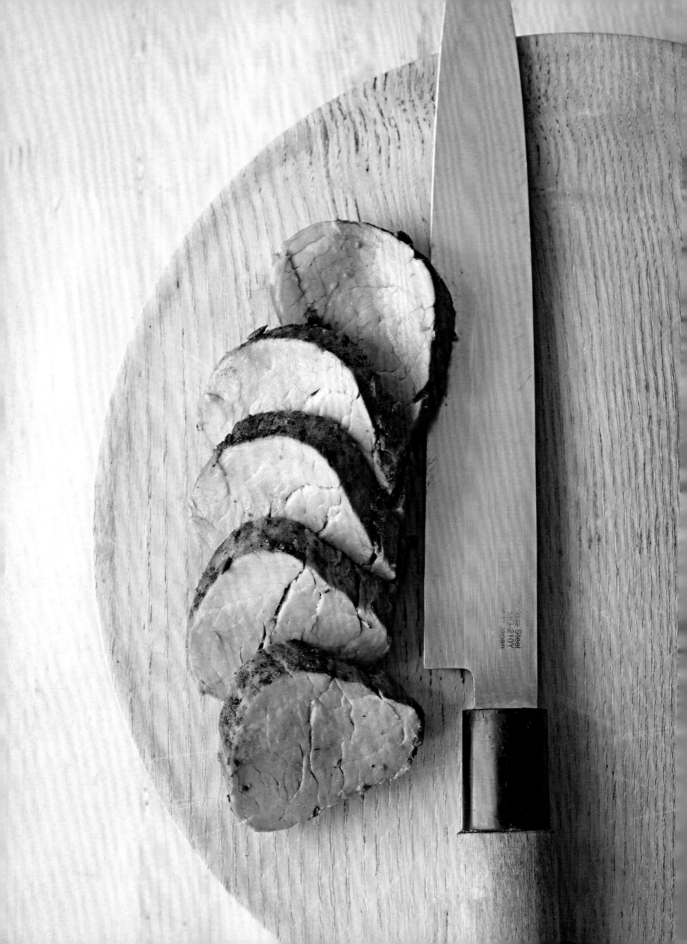

P Fillet of pork marinated with mustard, apple & sage

The lean pork is made especially delicious by the naturally sweet marinade that tenderizes the meat. Fennel seeds lend their distinctive flavour, adding phytosterols and antioxidants. This recipe may be served hot or cold with blanched salads for a satisfying take-to-work lunch.

Serves 4

500g (1lb 2oz) pork fillet (tenderloin)
20g (¾oz/1 tbsp) clarified butter

For the marinade:

80g (3oz) Granny Smith apples, cored and roughly chopped
8g (⅓oz) fresh sage leaves
1½ tbsp English mustard
2 tbsp maple syrup
pinch of salt
1 tsp fennel seeds, toasted
1 tbsp cider vinegar
2 tbsp water

To make the marinade, blitz all the ingredients in a blender until smooth. Cut the pork into 1cm (½in) slices and place them in a dish. Pour the marinade over them, then cover and leave to marinate in the fridge for at least 4 hours, preferably overnight.

To cook, heat the butter in a frying pan over a high heat and fry the pork medallions for about 2 minutes on each side. Brush with a little more marinade during cooking. Remove from the pan and leave to rest for 5 minutes.

Serve the pork with some roasted walnuts and crisp romaine lettuce tossed in Roasted red pepper, tomato, garlic & paprika dressing (see page 213).

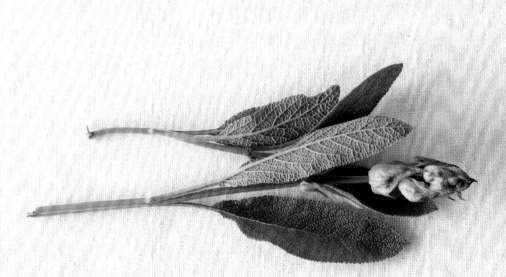

Ⓟ Porchetta with plum & fig chutney

Pork is an excellent form of animal protein on the Plan. Instead of just roasting a joint of pork, use this classic combination of herbs and spices to perfectly complement the chutney. Slowly cooking the pork belly in this way renders all the delicious flavour from the fat and the spices throughout the meat.

Serves 8

1kg (2lb 3½oz) pork belly, boned and skin scored

For the marinade:

25g (1oz) garlic, crushed

1 tsp fennel seeds, toasted and crushed in a pestle and mortar

2 tsp coriander seeds, toasted and crushed in a pestle and mortar

1 tbsp chopped lemon thyme leaves

1 tbsp chopped fresh rosemary leaves

grated zest of 1 lemon

pinch of pink Himalayan salt

1 tsp extra virgin olive oil

For the plum & fig chutney:

10g (½oz) coconut oil

100g (3½oz) shallots, finely chopped

1 garlic clove, grated

10g (½oz) fresh root ginger, peeled and grated

2 fresh red chillies, deseeded and finely chopped

2 star anise

1 cinnamon stick

2 tbsp cider vinegar

2 tbsp local runny honey

200g (7oz) plums, stoned and each cut into 8 pieces

150g (5oz) fresh figs, diced into 1cm (½in) pieces

Preheat the oven to 170°C, 325°F, Gas mark 3.

In a mixing bowl, mix all the ingredients for the marinade. Place the pork belly, skin-side down, on a board and massage the marinade into the meat. Roll the pork up tightly, skin outside, and tie securely with string ready for roasting. Place in a roasting pan.

Roast the pork in the preheated oven for 3 hours, basting it occasionally to make the crackling crisp and golden brown.

Meanwhile, make the chutney. Heat a small non-aluminium pan over a medium heat. Add the coconut oil and sweat the shallots for 2 minutes, then add the garlic, ginger, chilli, star anise and cinnamon. Reduce the heat and cook for 3–4 minutes.

Add the cider vinegar and honey. Turn up the heat and reduce by one-third, then add the plums and cook, covered with a lid, for 40 minutes over a really low heat. When the chutney is syrupy, add the figs and cook gently for a further 10–15 minutes.

Remove from the heat and allow to cool. (I like to leave the whole star anise and cinnamon stick in the chutney, rather than removing them, to improve the flavour.)

Allow the crisp pork belly to rest for at least 20 minutes before carving it into slices. Serve warm with the chutney.

CHEF'S TIP

This is a fresh chutney; store it in the fridge in an airtight container for up to one week.

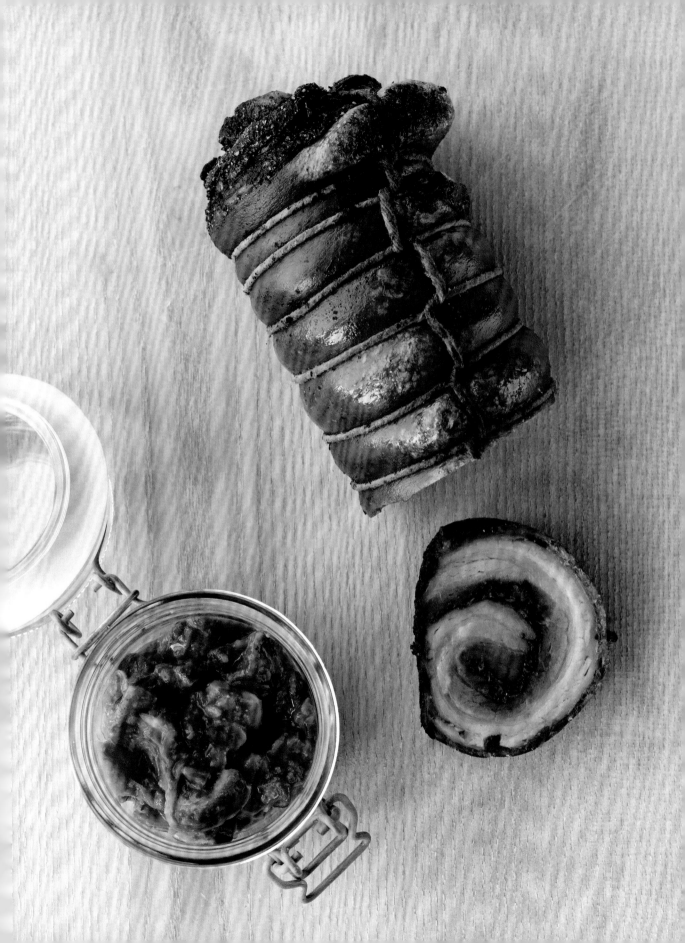

(P) Lamb koftas with tomato & onion salad

This is a brilliant way of using lamb as an alternative to minced (ground) beef. The koftas can be made in batches and freeze well, but you must reheat them thoroughly. Eat them cold for packed lunches and picnics. They are a good source of energy and digestion-healing amino acids.

Serves 4

500g (1lb 2oz) minced (ground) lean lamb

1 small onion, finely grated

1 fresh red chilli, deseeded and finely chopped

10g (½oz) fresh root ginger, peeled and grated

10g (½oz) mint leaves, chopped

10g (½oz) coriander (cilantro) leaves, chopped

½ tbsp ground cumin

½ tbsp ground coriander

2 garlic cloves, crushed

large pinch of salt

4 tsp melted clarified butter

squeeze of lemon juice

For the tomato & onion salad:

4 tomatoes

1 red onion, chopped

4 mint sprigs, chopped

2 coriander (cilantro) sprigs, chopped

1 tbsp olive oil

salt and ground black pepper

Make the koftas: mix together the minced (ground) lamb, onion, chilli, ginger, herbs, ground spices, garlic and salt in a bowl. Divide the mixture into 8 portions and roll each one into a long sausage shape. Thread each kofta onto a metal or bamboo skewer. Cover and keep in the fridge until you're ready to cook them.

To make the salad, chop the tomatoes and mix them with the onion, mint, coriander (cilantro) and olive oil. Season to taste.

When you're ready to cook the koftas, heat a griddle pan over a medium heat. Lightly brush the koftas with the clarified butter and cook them for 3–4 minutes on each side. Remove from the pan and set aside to rest for 10 minutes.

Serve the koftas on top of the tomato and onion salad, with a squeeze of lemon juice.

NUTRITION FACTS

Grass-fed lamb is packed with CLA (conjugated linoleic acid), which helps break down stored fats in the body. It may help to lower cholesterol and blood pressure, reducing inflammation in the gut and encouraging weight loss.

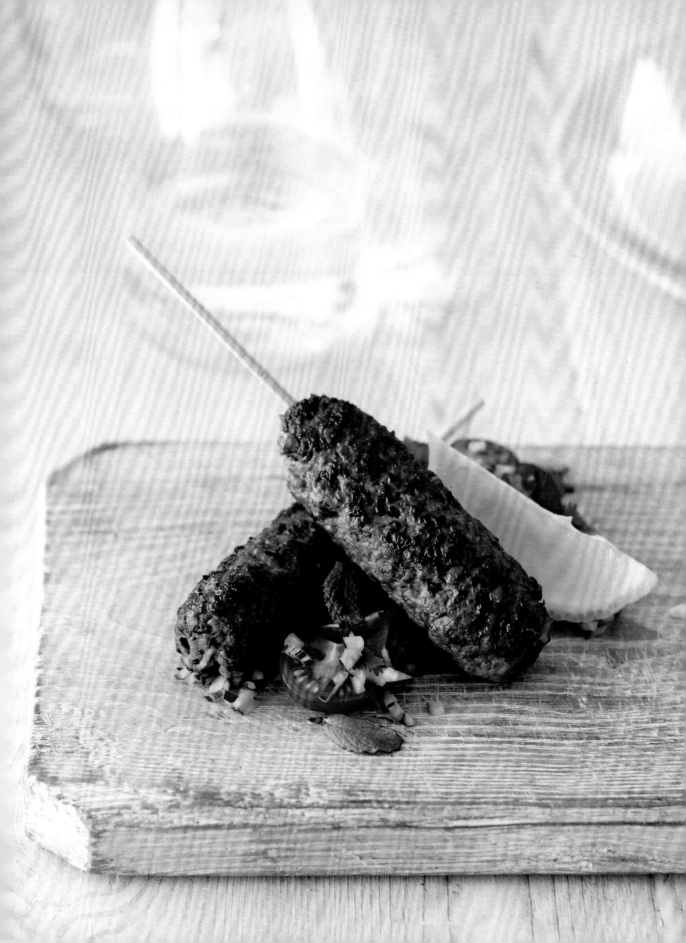

Marinated chicken breast with paprika, rosemary & lemon

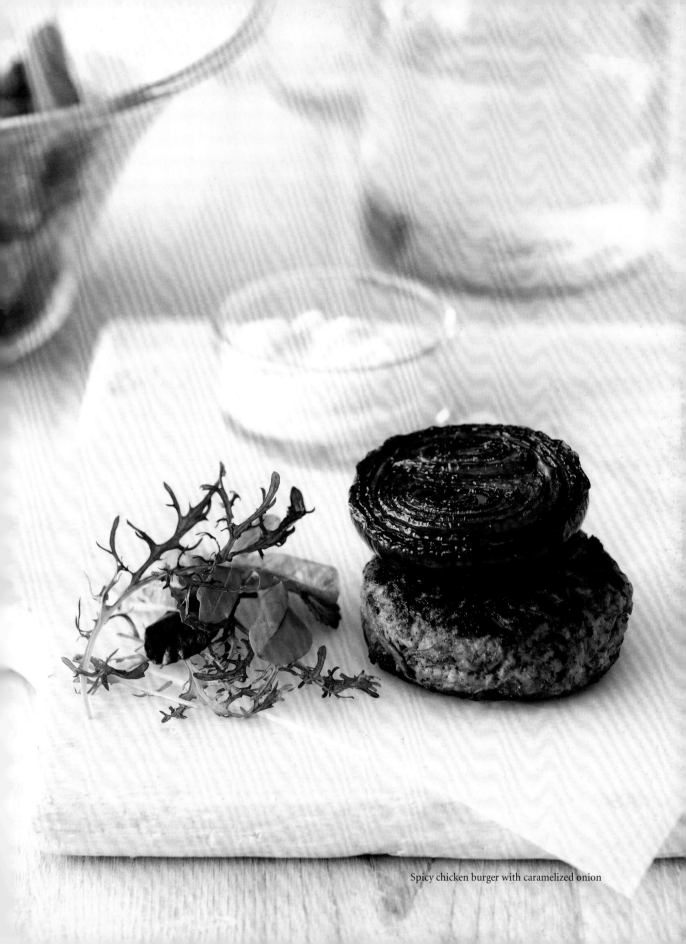

Spicy chicken burger with caramelized onion

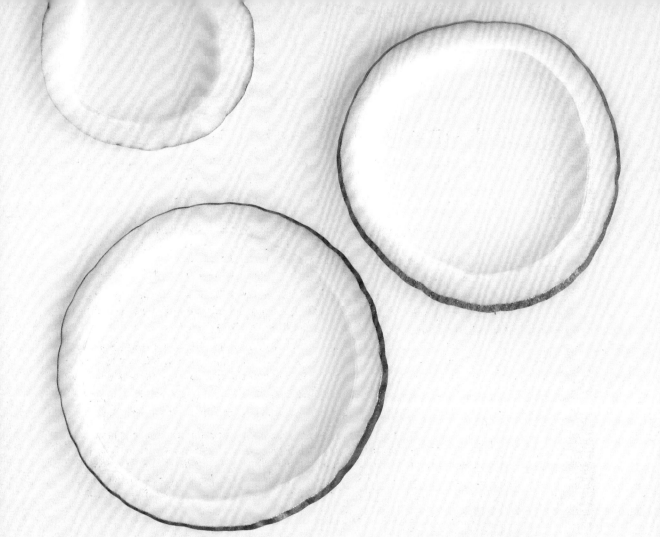

P Marinated chicken breast with paprika, rosemary & lemon

The best part about marinating is that it infuses meat and poultry with additional flavours and tenderizes the flesh, making it easier to break down in the gut. Chicken forms a large part of the protein offerings of the Plan, as it offers all the immune-boosting nutrients needed.

Serves 4

400g (14oz) skinned and boned chicken breast, cut into large chunks

2 tbsp melted clarified butter

For the marinade:

1½ tsp smoked paprika

2 garlic cloves, peeled

grated zest of 1 lemon

leaves stripped from a few fresh rosemary sprigs

2 tbsp lemon juice

pinch of salt

25g (1oz) Medjool dates, stoned and chopped

ground black pepper

75ml (3fl oz/scant ⅓ cup) water

To make the marinade, liquidize all the ingredients until smooth. Place the chicken strips in a bowl and pour the marinade over them. Massage it into the chicken, then cover and leave to marinate in the fridge for at least 4 hours or overnight.

Remove the chicken from the marinade and brush with the melted clarified butter. Cook on a hot griddle pan over a high heat for about 5 minutes on each side until cooked right through.

Illustrated on page 126.

P Spicy chicken burger with caramelized onion

Everyone loves a good burger, and these are simple to make and can be batch-frozen for last-minute meals. Prepare up to 'refrigerate until ready to cook' and then freeze the uncooked burgers. The recipe can also be used to make meatballs, which can be cooked and taken to work in place of falafels.

Serves 4

15g (½oz/1 tbsp) clarified butter plus extra melted for brushing

1 large onion, chopped

3 garlic cloves, crushed

2 tbsp chopped fresh thyme

2 fresh chillies, deseeded and chopped

750g (1lb 10 oz/3¼ cups) finely minced (ground) chicken breast

200g (7oz) carrot, coarsely grated

1 organic free-range egg, beaten

melted clarified butter for brushing

For the dry spice mix:

pinch of ground cumin

8g (⅓oz) ground coriander

pinch of ground allspice

pinch of ground nutmeg

good pinch of sea salt

ground black pepper

For the caramelized red onions:

2 small red onions, peeled and halved

15g (½oz/1 tbsp) clarified butter

pinch of Tangerine,cumin, fennel & chipotlc salt (see page 36)

For the cashew & garlic mayonnaise:

80g (3oz/1 cup) soaked cashew nuts
2 garlic cloves, roasted

1 organic free-range egg yolk

2 tsp cider vinegar

6 tbsp extra-virgin olive oil

pinch of mustard powder

salt and ground black pepper

Make the burgers: place a thick-bottomed pan over a medium heat. Melt the clarified butter and gently cook the onion, garlic, thyme and chillies until golden brown. Add the dry spice mix and cook for a further 5 minutes. Remove from the heat and allow to cool.

When the mixture is cool, mix together with the minced (ground) chicken, carrot and egg. Divide the mixture into 8 portions and shape into burgers. Refrigerate until ready to cook.

Make the caramelized red onions: melt the butter in a small pan set over a low heat. Add the onions and fry very gently for 10–15 minutes until they caramelize and turn golden. Sprinkle with the seasoned salt.

Make the cashew and garlic mayonnaise: put all the ingredients in a jug blender and blitz until smooth. Transfer to a serving bowl.

To cook the burgers, heat a ridged griddle pan over a medium heat. Brush the burgers with the melted clarified butter and cook for 4–5 minutes on each side until they are thoroughly cooked through. Check that the juices run clear when you push a skewer into the centre. Serve topped with the red onions with the cashew and garlic mayonnaise.

Illustrated on page 127.

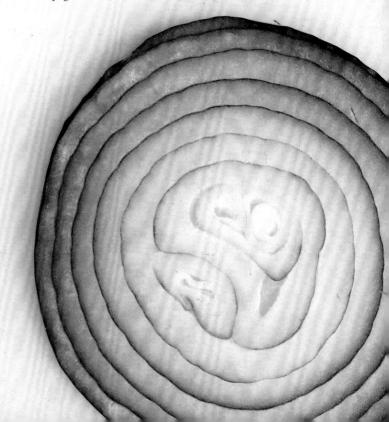

(P) Roasted tamarind, chilli, ginger & coriander chicken

The sweet and sour, spicy marinade should form more of a paste than a dressing, as the texture permeates the chicken flesh more effectively this way. It can also be used for roasting pork and beef. If wished, you can substitute poussins for individual servings with more visual impact.

Serves 4

1 x 1.5kg (3lb 5oz) roasting chicken

For the marinade:

30g (1¼oz) tamarind

2 peeled garlic cloves

1 fresh chilli, deseeded and chopped

12g (½oz) fresh root ginger, peeled and grated

1 tsp coriander seeds

½ tsp cumin seeds

1 tsp paprika

1 tbsp local runny honey

1 tbsp Tamari

1½ tsp sesame oil

5 tsp lemon juice

15g (½oz) fresh coriander (cilantro)

To spatchcock a chicken, place the chicken, breast-side down, on a chopping board. Using a sharp knife or scissors, cut along the back bone on either side to remove it. Turn the chicken over and press it out flat. Cut some score lines on each side of the chicken breasts ready for the marinade. Skewer with 2 bamboo skewers through the leg and breast to keep the flat shape.

Place all the marinade ingredients in a large jug and blend with a hand blender until the mixture forms a paste. Rub the paste into both sides of the chicken, working it in well with your hands to maximize the flavour.

Place the chicken on a non-stick baking tray lined with parchment paper. Cover and leave to marinate in the fridge for at least 2 hours, preferably overnight.

Preheat the oven to 180°C, 350°F, Gas mark 4.

Roast the chicken in the preheated oven for 50–60 minutes until cooked through and golden brown. Alternatively, it tastes great cooked over hot coals on a barbecue.

NUTRITION FACTS

Tamarind is derived from the fruit pod of the Asian tamarind tree, providing potent antioxidants and non-starch polysaccharides, which are allowed in the Plan as they are easy on a resting digestive system.

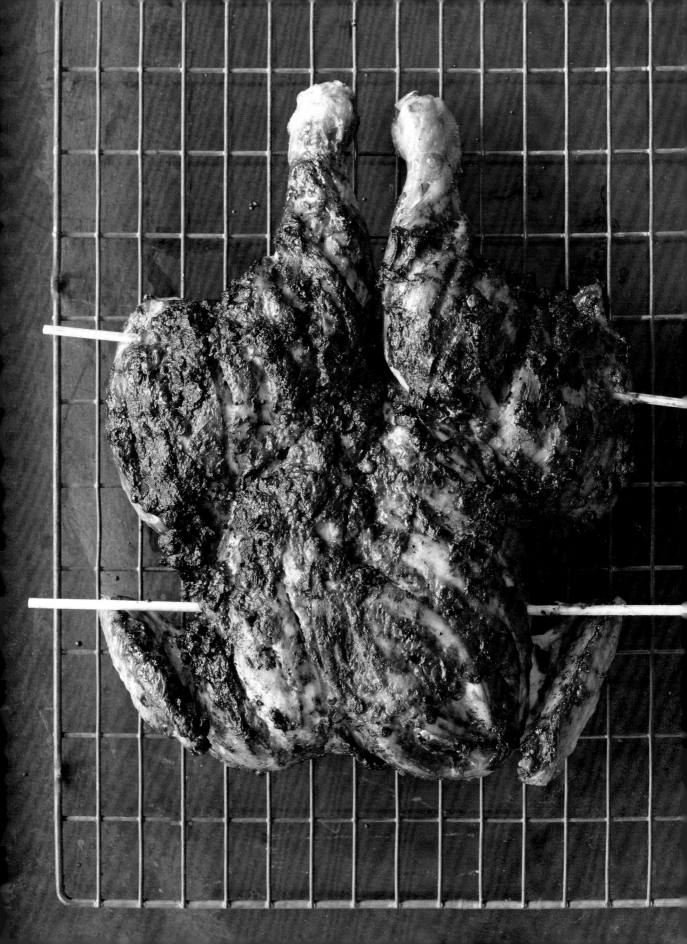

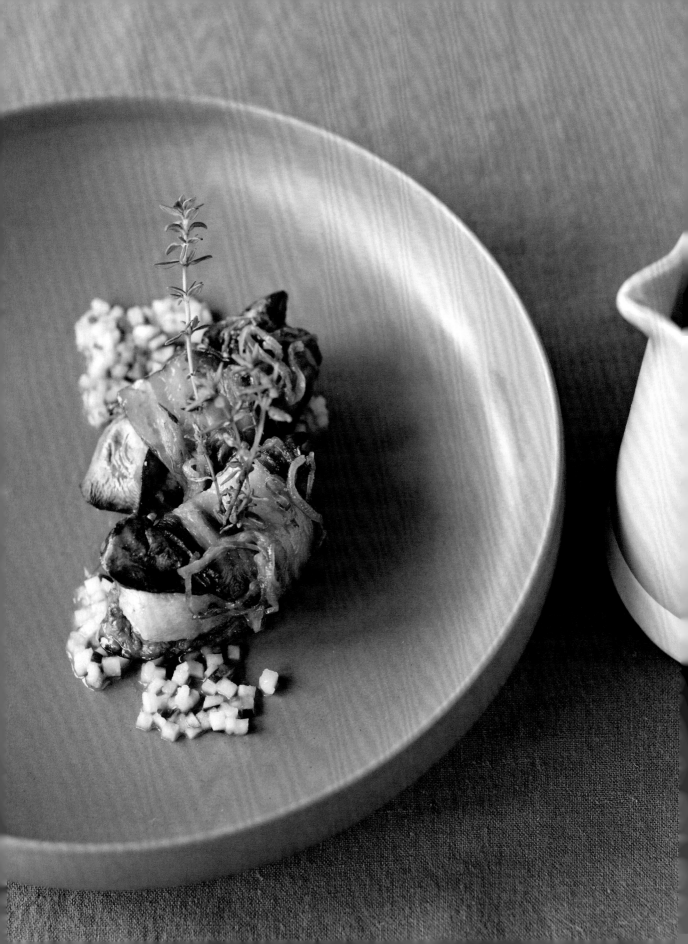

(P) Chicken livers with apple, pancetta & caramelized shallots

Forget chicken liver parfait and try this – it's a great way of eating an undervalued but fabulous food. The preparation may seem fiddly but it's worth it. Chicken livers are inexpensive and packed with iron, zinc and B vitamins to provide energy and support the immune system.

Serves 4

8 chicken livers, cleaned

1 Braeburn apple

8 slices pancetta (see page 69)

8 thyme sprigs, trimmed for use as skewers

salt and ground black pepper

olive oil for drizzling

For the caramelized shallots:

10g (½oz) coconut oil

80g (3oz) shallots, finely sliced

1 tbsp chopped fresh thyme leaves

1 tbsp sherry vinegar

80ml (3fl oz/scant ⅓ cup) apple juice

For the apple mustard vinaigrette:

60g (2½oz) red apple, cored and cut into 3mm (⅛in) dice

1 tsp English mustard

2 tsp apple cider vinegar

1 tsp local runny honey

3 tbsp olive oil

Preheat the oven to 170°C, 325°F, Gas mark 3.

Remove any sinews from the chicken livers. Peel and core the apple, and cut it into 8 wedges.

Place a slice of pancetta on a chopping board. Lay a chicken liver and a wedge of apple at one end of the pancetta and roll up the entire length. Skewer with a thyme sprig through the centre of the apple and chicken liver to secure them, and repeat with the remaining chicken livers, apple wedges and pancetta.

Arrange on a non-stick baking tray ready for cooking and season with salt and pepper. Drizzle a little olive oil over the top.

In a small pan set over a medium heat, melt the coconut oil and add the shallots. Cook until the shallots are softened and golden brown. Add the thyme, sherry vinegar and apple juice, then turn up the heat and reduce until the shallots are sticky. Keep warm.

Make the apple mustard vinaigrette by mixing all the ingredients together in a small bowl.

Cook the chicken liver skewers in the preheated oven for about 14 minutes until the pancetta is crisp and golden and the livers are cooked. Serve the chicken livers with the shallots and apple mustard vinaigrette.

CHEF'S TIP

Don't overcook the chicken livers as they will become bitter. Chop the apple for the vinaigrette finely to release its sweetness.

P Shredded pheasant salad with pickled mushrooms

Pheasant has a reputation for being dry but this is wonderfully moist. Although the meat is lean, it is full of flavour and density. The pickled mushrooms provide the extra digestive ingredient in this dish as well as spice – perfect as a take-to-work salad.

Serves 4

500ml (17fl oz/2 cups) Chicken Broth (see page 44)

4 pheasant breasts, skinned and boned

1 tbsp coconut oil

8 baby gem lettuce leaves

40g (1½oz) Preserved Pickled Mushrooms (see page 151)

For the vinaigrette dressing:

few tarragon sprigs, finely chopped

10g (½oz) flat-leaf parsley, finely chopped

10g (½oz) chives, finely chopped

10g (½oz) chervil, finely chopped

1 shallot, diced

4 tsp cider vinegar

2 tbsp extra virgin olive oil

1 tbsp local runny honey

juice of ½ lemon

sea salt and black pepper

To make the vinaigrette, whisk all the ingredients together in a large bowl ready to marinate the pheasant later.

In a medium-sized pan, bring the chicken broth to a gentle simmer. Set a large frying pan over a high heat and add the coconut oil. When it starts to smoke, add the pheasant and fry for 2 minutes on each side until golden brown.

Transfer the pheasant to a chopping board and shred thinly. Mix with the vinaigrette dressing and set aside to cool. The pheasant should be slightly pink when it's shredded but it will continue to cook in the dressing.

When cool, cover the pheasant and keep in the fridge for up to 3 days. This will taste better the day after it's made.

Serve at room temperature with baby gem lettuce leaves and a few pickled mushrooms on top.

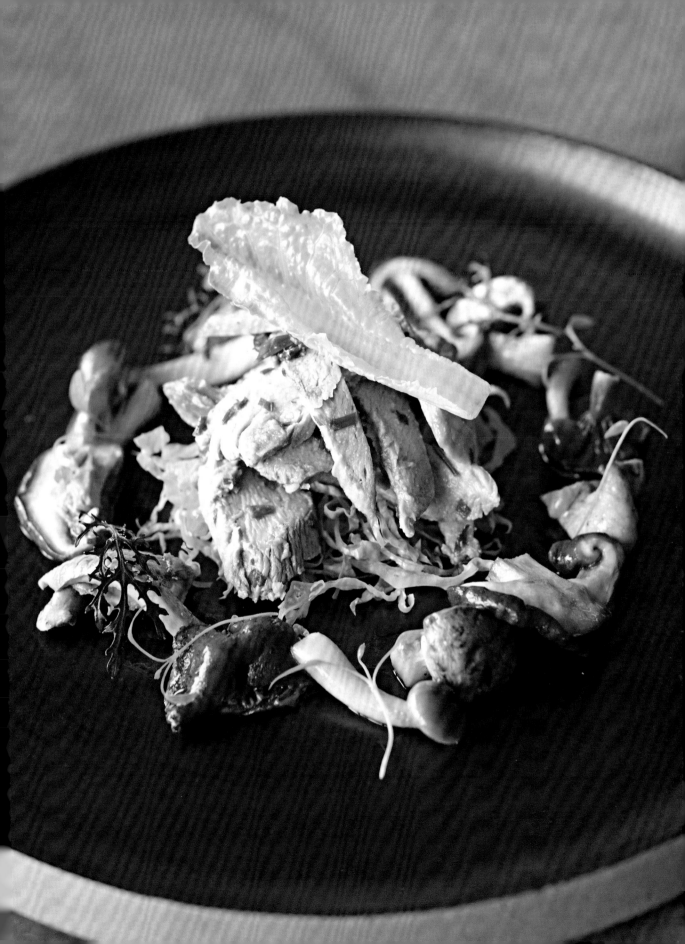

P Escabeche of red mullet

This is a great dish to cook in advance as the flavour continues to develop as it cools. Rather than overcooking the fish, allow the spices, herbs and orange sauce to 'cook' the dish during the 'standing' process. This is the secret to maintaining the fish's texture and moisture.

Serves 4

½ tsp allspice berries

1 star anise

½ tsp coriander seeds

½ tsp pink peppercorns

4 tsp groundnut oil

4 large or 8 small red mullet fillets, bones removed and skin scored

1 small onion, finely sliced

100g (3½oz) fennel bulb, finely sliced

1 carrot, finely sliced

1 garlic clove, finely sliced

2 thyme sprigs

750ml (1¼ pints/3 cups) water

100ml (3½fl oz/generous ⅓ cup) cider vinegar

1 tsp grated orange zest

pinch of salt

2 bay leaves

1 fresh orange, peeled and cut horizontally into 8 slices

In a spice grinder, grind the allspice, star anise and coriander seeds, then lightly toast them in a small frying pan over a medium heat. Watch them to make sure they don't catch and burn. Remove from the heat and add the pink peppercorns.

In a large frying pan, heat the groundnut oil, then place the mullet, skin-side down, in the hot pan. Cook for 30 seconds to sear the skin, then remove from the pan and place in a dish.

Add the onion, fennel, carrot and garlic to the hot pan and cook for 5 minutes. Add the toasted spice mixture and cook until golden. Add the thyme, water, cider vinegar, orange zest, salt and bay leaves. Bring to the boil and cook rapidly to reduce by half.

Lay the orange slices on the mullet fillets and spoon over the sauce and vegetables. Completely cover the dish with cling film (plastic wrap). Serve warm after 30 minutes or allow to cool completely and serve cold. This will keep in the fridge for up to 3 days.

NUTRITION FACTS

Red mullet is one of the unsung heroes of the fish world. As well as being packed with flavour it is rich in anti-inflammatory Omega-3, which helps with gut healing, mood regulation, and skin and hair quality.

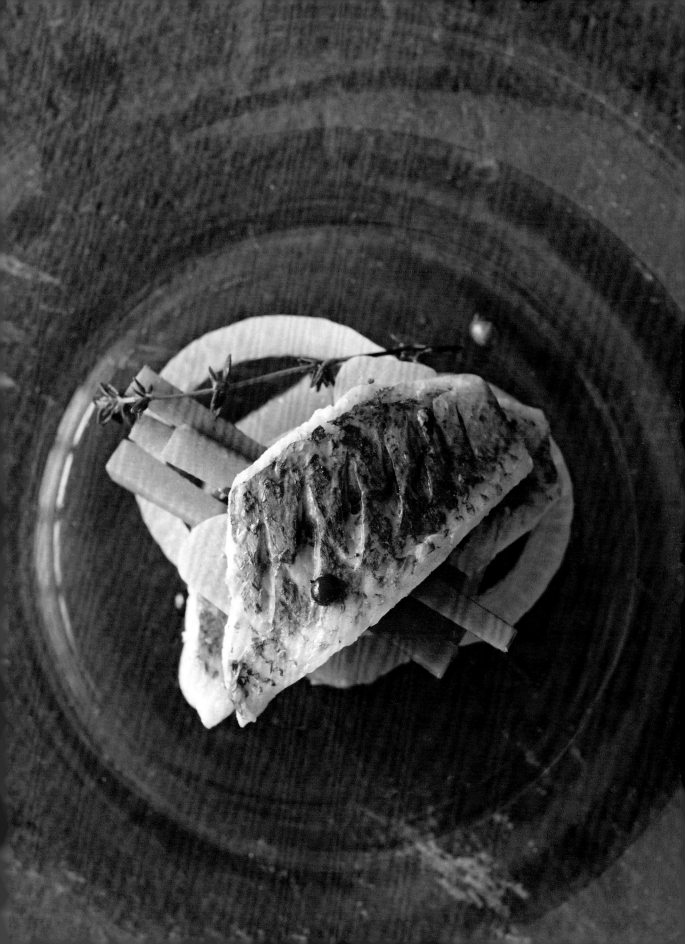

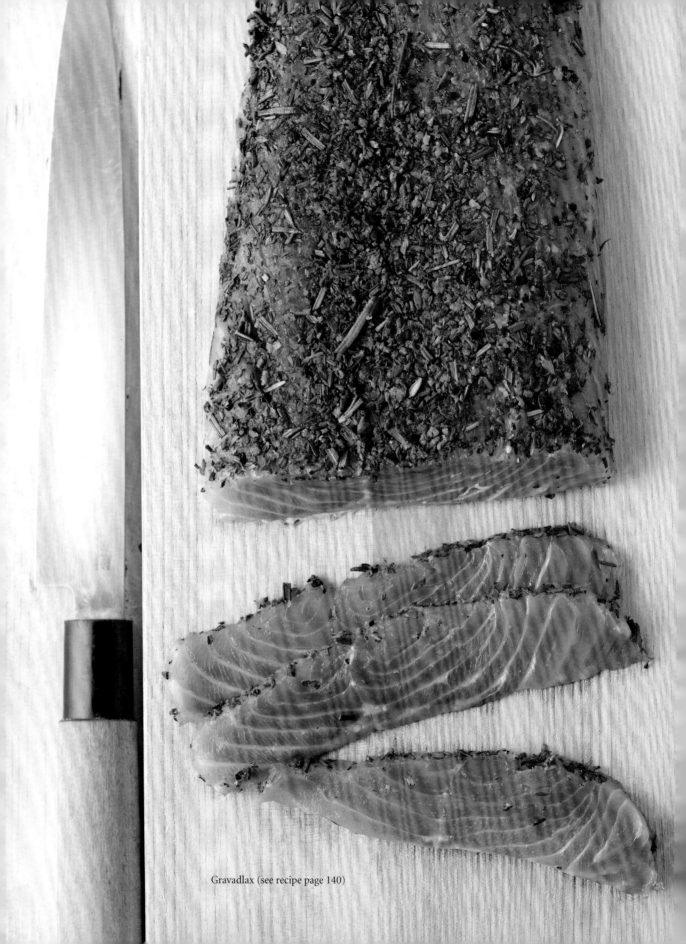

Gravadlax (see recipe page 140)

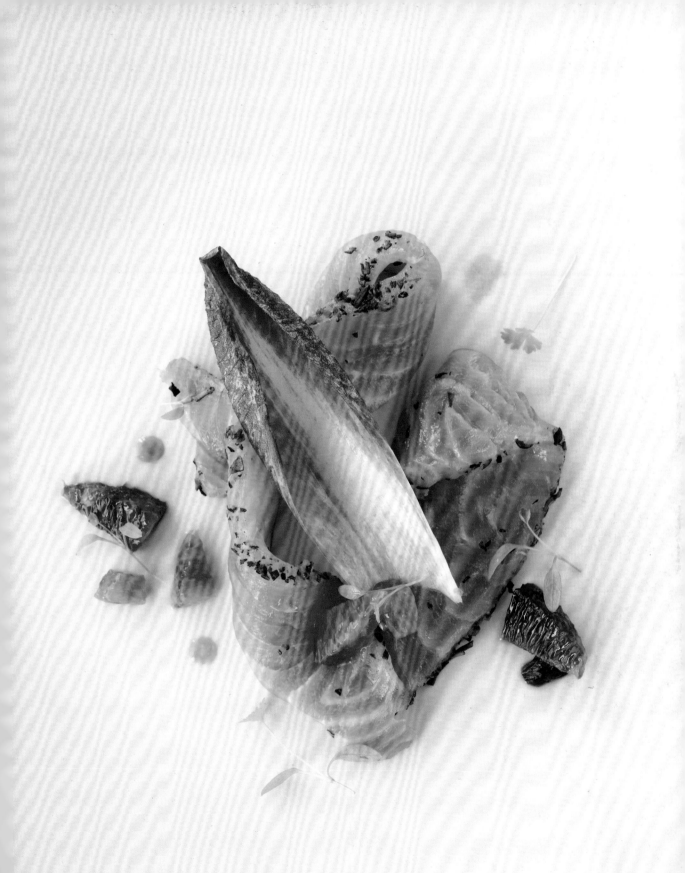

Gravadlax with tarragon, juniper, ginger & orange

(P) Gravadlax with tarragon, juniper, ginger & orange

This sweet-and-sour alternative for the classic dish from Scandinavia has a smörgasbord of flavours. Traditionally, gravadlax requires too much sugar to be considered on this Plan, but the maple syrup creates a natural sweetness that contributes to the marinating of the fish.

Serves 12

10g (½oz) juniper berries

10g (½oz) coriander seeds

15g (½oz) tarragon leaves

15g (½oz) orange zest, grated

25g (1oz) salt

4cm (1¾in) piece fresh root ginger, peeled and grated

2 tbsp maple syrup

1kg (2lb 3½oz) salmon fillet, skin on and pin boned

For the blood orange & chicory (Belgian endive) salad:

3 blood oranges

2 tbsp chia oil

salt and ground black pepper

1 tsp local runny honey

1 head red chicory (Belgian endive)

Using a pestle and mortar, grind the juniper berries and coriander seeds to a paste. Add the tarragon and orange zest and grind a little more, then mix in the salt and ginger to make the curing paste.

Place the salmon fillet, skin-side down, on a piece of non-stick baking parchment and rub the curing paste into the flesh of the salmon to cover it thinly. Fold the parchment over the top, then wrap tightly in several layers of cling film (plastic wrap).

Place the wrapped salmon fillet on a tray and then weigh it down with a heavy weight. Leave in the fridge for a couple of days before turning it over and weighing the other side down. Put it back in the fridge to cure for a further 2 days. When the salmon is ready, it should be firm to the touch.

Just before serving, make the salad. Peel and segment the blood oranges over a small bowl to catch the juice. Whisk the chia oil, some salt and pepper and the honey with the juice and drizzle over the chicory (Belgian endive) leaves and orange segments.

Remove the cling film (plastic wrap) and parchment paper from the salmon and carefully scrape off the curing mixture with the back of a knife – it's a little bitter if left on. Slice the salmon very thinly and serve on the dressed blood orange and chicory (Belgian endive) salad.

Illustrated on pages 138/9.

P Snapper ceviche with avocado & pomelo

This is a good way of enjoying fish at its freshest. Snapper is light yet firm, and the lime, ginger and chilli marinade enlivens its taste. Pomelo, one of the largest citrus fruits, complements the snapper perfectly. This is a wonderfully sophisticated yet simply-prepared dish.

Serves 4

10g (½oz) fresh root ginger, peeled and finely diced

1–2 limes, juiced

1 tsp local runny honey

pinch of sea salt

80g (3oz) pomelo, peeled and broken into pistils

1 fresh green chilli, deseeded and finely chopped

250g (8oz) fresh snapper fillets, skinned and boned

1 tbsp olive oil

1 tbsp chopped coriander (cilantro)

1 tbsp chopped mint

1 small ripe avocado, peeled, stoned and sliced

3 red spring onions (scallions), chopped

baby coriander (cilantro) leaves to garnish

In a large non-aluminium bowl, mix the ginger, lime juice, honey, salt, pomelo and chilli. Slice the snapper fillets really thinly, then add to the lime mixture with the olive oil.

Cover the bowl and leave in the fridge for 15–20 minutes. Stir after 5 minutes. You will know when the fish is ready as it will have turned opaque and 'cooked' in the lime juice.

Remove the bowl from the fridge, strain the fish in a colander and stir in the fresh coriander (cilantro) and mint.

Serve the sliced snapper on a plate, garnished with slices of avocado, a sprinkle of spring onions (scallions) and a few baby coriander (cilantro) leaves.

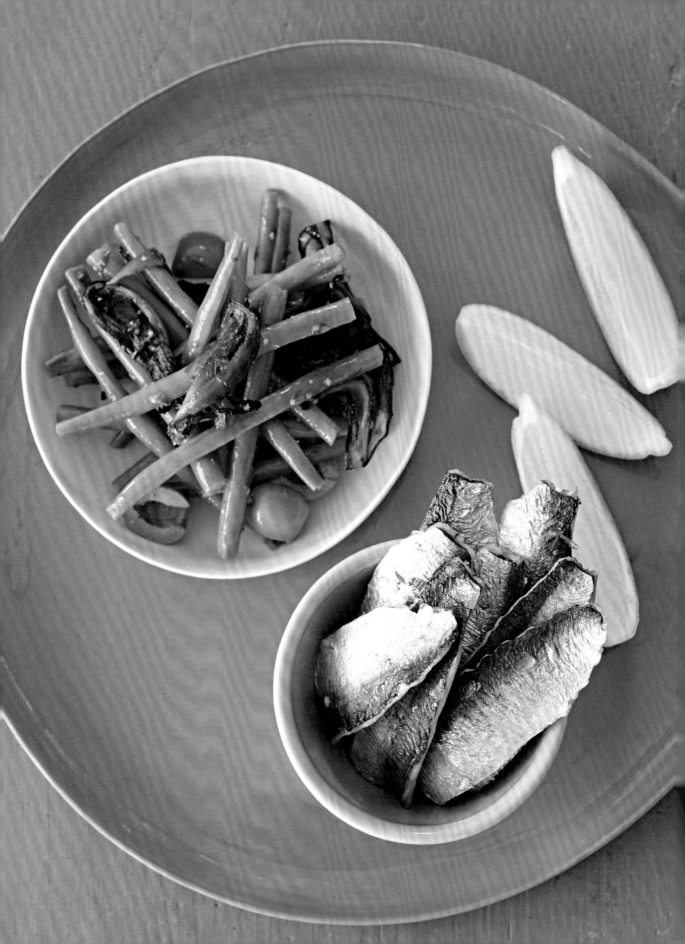

P Sardine fillets with green beans, roasted red onions & olives

The green beans and onions cut through the oiliness of the sardines, which are packed with healthy Omega-3 yet seldom cooked fresh. Nothing beats the taste of fresh sardines – they are readily available in most fishmongers and the fresh fish counters of many supermarkets.

Serves 4

100g (3½oz) fine green beans
1 tsp coriander seeds
1 tsp melted coconut oil
1 large red onion, peeled, halved and cut into 16 wedges
60g (2½oz) green olives
8 sardines, filleted and scaled
1 lemon, cut into wedges to serve

For the dressing:

1 tbsp wholegrain mustard
4 tsp extra virgin olive oil
1 tbsp cider vinegar
1 tsp lemon juice
5g (¼oz) capers, chopped
1 tsp chopped thyme leaves
1 tbsp chopped parsley
sea salt and ground black pepper

Preheat the oven to 180°C, 350°F, Gas mark 4.

Bring a small pan of water to the boil and blanch the green beans for 2 minutes, then refresh under cold running water to cool.

Crush the coriander seeds in a pestle and mortar. Mix them with the melted coconut oil and gently toss the red onion wedges in this mixture. Arrange them on a non-stick baking tray and roast in the preheated oven for about 10 minutes until golden brown.

To make the dressing, whisk all the ingredients together, seasoning to taste with salt and pepper. In a large mixing bowl, toss the cooked beans, roasted onions and olives in the dressing. Leave for up to 1 hour before serving.

Place the sardines on a non-stick baking tray and simply roast them in the preheated oven for 10 minutes. Serve on top of the dressed beans, onions and olives with the lemon wedges.

NUTRITION FACTS

The anti-inflammatory essential fats in this dish will help to calm the most troubled digestive system. The dressing alleviates the oiliness of the fish, and the two can be combined into a milder-tasting dip or pâté.

Marinated grilled mackerel
with fennel, coriander & lemon

Grilled sole fillets marinated in
ginger & tangerine juice

P Marinated grilled mackerel with fennel, coriander & lemon

Fresh mackerel is almost unbeatable for flavour and texture. The beauty of this dish is the marinade, which can be made in advance, as the taste develops with age. This is an incredibly easy dish to prepare and it can be adapted for use with other fish of your choice.

Serves 4

4 small whole mackerel, cleaned, gutted and scored with a sharp knife

2 tbsp clarified butter

2 lemons, cut in half

For the marinade:

1 garlic clove, roughly chopped

2 tsp coriander seeds, toasted in a dry pan

2 tsp fennel seeds, toasted in a dry pan

finely grated zest of ½ lemon

1 tbsp oregano leaves stripped from stalks

1 tbsp local runny honey

1 tbsp lemon juice

2 spring onions (scallions), sliced

1 tbsp dried rose petals

pinch of salt

To make the marinade, liquidize all the ingredients until smooth. Score some deep cuts down the length of the mackerel with a sharp knife, then place them in a large dish and pour the marinade over the top. Massage the marinade into the cuts along each fish, then cover and leave to marinate in the fridge for 1 hour.

Just before cooking, remove the mackerel from the marinade and brush with clarified butter. Cook them under a hot grill or over hot coals on a barbecue for about 6–8 minutes on each side. Brush occasionally with butter and any leftover marinade.

Cook the lemons, cut-side down, in a ridged griddle pan over a high heat for a few minutes until starting to brown. Serve them immediately with the grilled mackerel.

Illustrated on page 144.

CHEF'S TIP

The flavour is all in the marinade. You can prepare it several days in advance if wished and then stored in a screwtop jar in the fridge until required.

P Grilled sole fillets marinated in ginger & tangerine juice

Tangerine and ginger are a marriage made in heaven — light enough to add sweetness and spice. Cooking it quickly preserves the nutritional content and delicate flavour of the lemon sole. This dish can be cooled and added to one of the blanched salads for an easy lunch.

Serves 4

4 x 125g (4oz) lemon sole fillets

2 tbsp melted clarified butter

20g (¾oz) butter (not clarified)

For the marinade:

20g (¾oz) fresh root ginger, peeled and roughly chopped

100ml (3½fl oz/generous ⅓ cup) tangerine juice, with some tangerine segments removed over a bowl for the butter

finely grated zest of 2 tangerines

½ tsp Chinese five-spice powder

1 tsp chopped thyme leaves

1 tbsp local runny honey

pinch of salt

2 tbsp water

To make the marinade, liquidize all the ingredients until smooth. Lay the sole fillets in a flat dish and pour the marinade over the top. Cover and leave to marinate in the fridge for 1 hour.

Place the sole fillets on a non-stick baking tray and brush with the melted clarified butter. Reserve the leftover marinade. Cook the sole under a preheated grill for 4–5 minutes on each side until cooked. If the fillets are thin, there is no need to turn them during cooking.

Just before serving, heat the butter in a pan. As it starts to turn brown, add the reserved tangerine segments and 2 tablespoons of the leftover marinade to the butter to stop it burning. Pour over the fish and serve immediately.

Illustrated on page 145.

(P) Spinach, butternut squash & lentil frittata

Eggs are a good protein choice, providing all the nutrients we need for healing and repair. Frittatas are useful dishes to prepare in advance, so there is always something in the fridge when you're hungry. This may be eaten at any time of the day and is a great food on-the-go.

Serves 4

20g (¾oz) coconut oil

60g (2½oz) shallots, finely sliced

1 tsp curry powder

100g (3½oz) butternut squash, peeled and grated

50g (2oz) courgette (zucchini), grated

50g (2oz/⅓ cup) cooked Puy lentils, drained

20g (¾oz) baby spinach leaves

2 spring onions (scallions), chopped

100ml (3½fl oz/generous ⅓ cup) almond milk

3 organic free-range eggs

salt and ground black pepper

7g (¼oz) coriander (cilantro), chopped

Preheat the oven to 200°C, 400°F, Gas mark 6.

In an ovenproof frying pan, melt the coconut oil and fry the shallots with the curry powder over a low heat until it is lightly browned. Stir continuously to prevent the curry powder burning. Add the butternut squash and cook, stirring, for 1 minute. Stir in the courgette (zucchini) and remove from the heat.

Allow to cool slightly, then add the Puy lentils, spinach and spring onions (scallions) and mix well.

In a blender, blend together the almond milk, eggs, some salt and pepper and the coriander (cilantro). Pour over the lentils and vegetables in the pan. Level the top, pushing it down with the back of a spoon, and bake in the preheated oven for 20 minutes.

Remove from the oven and unmould on to a serving plate. Serve immediately with the Roasted cherry tomatoes (see below).

(P) Roasted cherry tomatoes with maple syrup & chilli

Sweet chilli sauce is the modern ketchup, and this is my version. It's so simple to make, there are no preservatives in it, you can make it in minutes, and it goes with almost everything.

Serves 4

1 large fresh red chilli, deseeded and chopped

50ml (2fl oz/scant ¼ cup) maple syrup

12 cherry tomatoes

Preheat the oven to 200°C, 400°F, Gas mark 6.

Bring a small pan of water to the boil. Blanch the chopped chilli for 1 minute. Remove and refresh under cold running water. Repeat twice more with fresh water, then drain.

In a blender, blend the maple syrup and chilli together. Pour over the cherry tomatoes in a baking dish or roasting pan and roast in the preheated oven for 8 minutes.

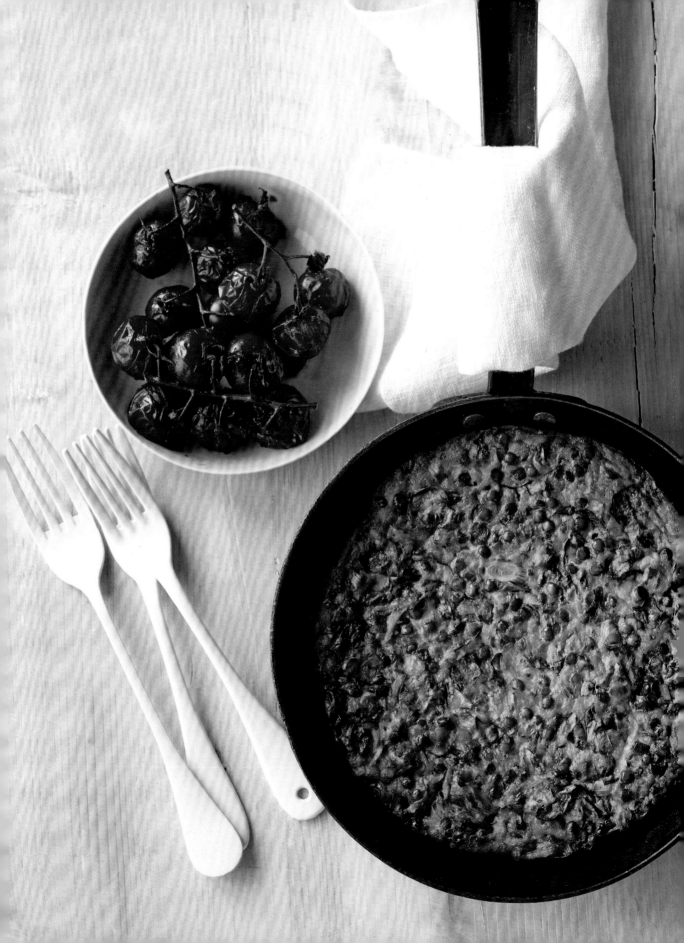

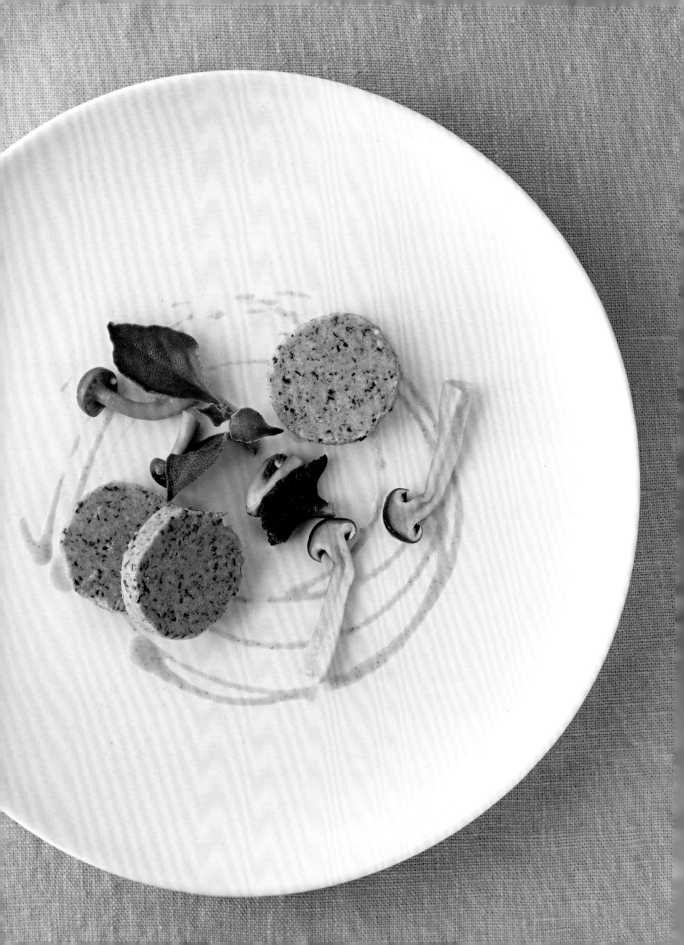

(P) Mushroom mousse with pickled mushrooms

Delicately flavoured shiitake is high in vegetarian protein and the best immune-boosting mushroom. This dish is good when you want something light, whilst still adhering to the principle of having protein with every meal. It can be cooked without the Madeira.

Serves 6

50g (2oz/¼ cup) unsalted butter

30g (1¼oz) shallots, sliced

1 garlic clove, sliced

1 tbsp thyme leaves

150g (5oz) shiitake mushrooms

100m (3½fl oz/generous ⅓ cup) water

70ml (3fl oz/scant ⅓ cup) Madeira

40g (1½oz) Preserved Pickled Mushrooms (see below)

lettuce leaves, to serve

Walnut, tarragon, shallot & honey dressing (see page 212)

Heat a frying pan over a medium heat. Melt 20g (1¾oz/2 tbsp) of the butter and fry the shallots until golden. Add the garlic and thyme and cook for 1 minute. Add the mushrooms and water.

Turn the heat down, cover with a lid and steam the mushrooms for 10 minutes. Uncover the pan and add the Madeira. Reduce over a high heat until the mushrooms are golden brown and the liquid has evaporated.

Put the mushroom mixture into a food processor and add the remaining butter. Blitz until smooth.

Place a large sheet of cling film (plastic wrap) on a board and spoon the mushroom mousse mixture on top. Roll up into a sausage shape, twisting the ends of the cling film (plastic wrap) to seal it.

Chill in the fridge for a couple of hours before slicing the mousse into 1cm (½in) slices. Arrange on serving plates and serve with pickled mushrooms (see below) and lettuce leaves drizzled with Walnut, tarragon, shallot and honey dressing.

(P) Preserved pickled mushrooms

Try this method of preparing fresh mushrooms, and add them to a range of cooked dishes and salads. The cooking brine really brings out their natural flavour and delicacy.

Serves 8

180g (6oz) wild mushrooms, e.g. shiitake, oyster, girolles, trompettes

For the brine:

150ml (¼ pint/⅔ cup) cider vinegar

250ml (8fl oz/1 cup) water

3 rosemary sprigs

1 tsp whole black peppercorns

6 bay leaves

4 whole cloves

2 medium shallots, sliced

2 garlic cloves, crushed

pinch of salt

500ml (16fl oz/2 cups) olive oil to cover

To make the cooking brine, boil the cider vinegar, water, rosemary, peppercorns, bay leaves, cloves, shallots, garlic and salt until the liquid has reduced by half. Remove from the heat.

Wash the mushrooms thoroughly, then blanch them in a pan of salted boiling water for 10 seconds. Refresh under cold running water before adding them to the warm reduced brine. Set aside until they cool to room temperature.

When cool, remove the mushrooms from the brine and drain thoroughly in a colander. Place the mushrooms in a sterilized preserving jar and cover with olive oil. Pop the lid on and keep in the fridge for up to one month.

Ⓟ Grilled asparagus with poached egg

Packed with energy-giving B vitamins, asparagus also stimulates the kidneys and possesses antibacterial properties. Griddling retains its crunchy texture, and adding eggs creates the best breakfast, brunch or supper. The al verde sauce yields additional iron-rich energy.

Serves 4

24 asparagus spears, tough stalks removed and peeled with a potato peeler

20g (¾oz/1½ tbsp) melted clarified butter

2 tsp cider vinegar

4 organic free-range eggs

For the al verde sauce:

80g (3oz) broccoli florets

30g (1oz) baby spinach leaves

few basil sprigs

30g (1oz/¼ cup) toasted hazelnuts

2 garlic cloves, toasted or roasted in the oven

50ml (2fl oz/scant ¼ cup) olive oil

salt and ground black pepper

Make the al verde sauce: blanch the broccoli in boiling water for 1 minute, then refresh under cold running water and drain well. Blend the broccoli with the other ingredients until smooth, using a stick blender. Add a little cold water until the sauce has the consistency of whipped cream.

Before cooking, roll the asparagus in the melted butter. Heat a ridged griddle pan over a high heat and place the asparagus carefully in the hot pan. Season with salt and pepper and place another pan or flat lid on top of the asparagus, so that it steams as well as grills. Cook for 1–2 minutes on each side, then remove.

Bring a pan of water to the boil. Add the vinegar and poach the eggs for 3 minutes.

Arrange the warm asparagus on serving plates with a spoonful of the al verde sauce and top with a poached egg.

Sprinkle a little sea salt and black pepper over the poached egg and serve immediately.

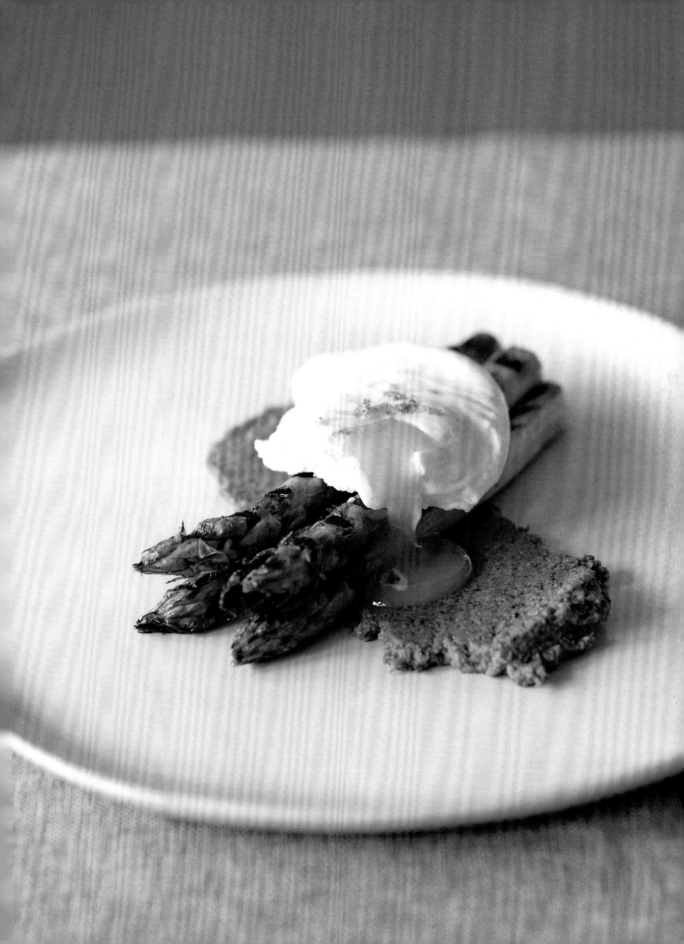

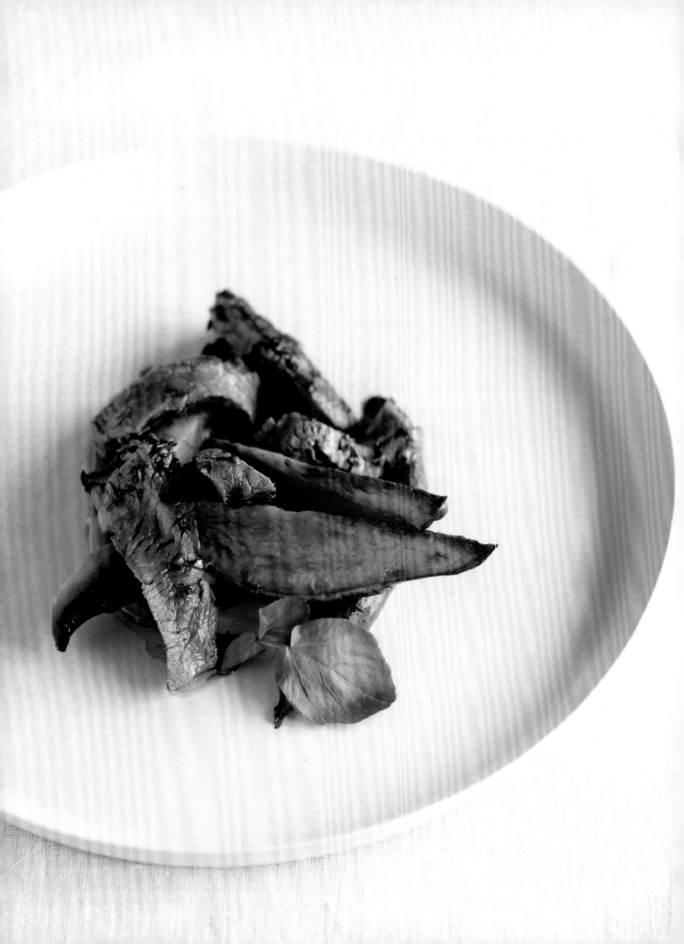

Post-Plan everyday meals

It may be that not all of the root vegetables, pulses and grains you can eat post-Plan appeal to you, but having the choice is the critical factor. Sweet potatoes, parsnips, amaranth, buckwheat, millet, quinoa, spelt and bulghur wheat give you more variety. The following dishes show you some additional ways in which these permitted post-Plan foods can open up your repertoire.

P+ Marinated rib-eye beef with sweet potato wedges

This marinade brings out the best of what is, arguably, the tastiest cut of grass-fed organic beef. Griddling the outside of the beef and allowing it to rest seals in the flavour and keeps it tender and succulent. Serve it cold with salad for lunch or to take it to work with you.

Serves 4

4 x 150g (5oz) rib-eye steaks

50ml (2fl oz/scant ¼ cup) clarified butter

watercress sprigs, to garnish

2 sliced flat mushrooms, grilled with melted butter

For the marinade:

few fresh thyme sprigs, leaves roughly chopped

2 tsp grated fresh horseradish root

1 garlic clove crushed

20g (¾oz) local runny honey

4 tsp Tamari

2 tbsp water

For the sweet potato wedges:

20g (¾oz/2 tbsp) butter

juice of 1 lemon

salt and ground black pepper

2 small sweet potatoes, washed and cut into 1cm (½in) thick wedges

To make the marinade, blitz all the ingredients in a blender until smooth. Place the rib-eye steaks in a dish and pour the marinade over the top. Cover and leave to marinate in the fridge for at least 4 hours, preferably overnight.

Preheat the oven to 190°C, 375°F, Gas mark 5.

Melt the butter for the sweet potatoes in a pan. Add the lemon juice and seasoning. Pour the seasoned melted butter over the sweet potatoes in a bowl and coat them thoroughly. Line a roasting tray with parchment paper and place the potatoes on top. Roast in the preheated oven for 20–25 minutes until cooked and golden.

Meanwhile, heat a griddle pan over a high heat and cook the rib-eye steaks for 1½ minutes on each side to seal them. Cook a little longer, depending on how well cooked you like them. Brush frequently with the marinade. Remove from the pan and leave to rest for 10 minutes.

Slice the steaks thinly and serve garnished with watercress sprigs and grilled mushrooms with the sweet potato wedges.

NUTRITION FACTS

Horseradish root is packed with antibacterial and antiviral properties, while the rib-eye beef delivers abundant protein as well as CLA (conjugated linoleic acid), which aids weight loss.

P+ Slow-roasted lamb with rose harissa & beans

Slow-roasting tenderizes the meat, locks in the moisture and allows the flavours to develop. You can buy harissa in a jar, but making it yourself is well worth the effort. This is a whole meal in itself with the butter (lima) beans. You can also eat it cold accompanied by a blanched salad.

Serves 6

300g (10oz/1 generous cup) dried butter (lima) beans, soaked in water with lemon juice overnight

1.5kg (3lb 5oz) shoulder of lamb, bone removed

1 large red onion, sliced

½ bunch of thyme

700ml (1 pint 3½fl oz/2¾ cups) Chicken Broth (see page 44)

salt and ground black pepper

For the rose harissa:

1 large red (bell) pepper

1 small onion, peeled

2 garlic cloves, unpeeled

olive oil for drizzling

½ tsp ground cumin

2 tbsp lemon juice

4 tsp cider vinegar

pinch of smoked paprika

½ tsp ground coriander

pinch of ground caraway

1 fresh red chilli, deseeded

60ml (2½fl oz/¼ cup) chia oil

2 tbsp chopped mint

1 tsp dried rose petals

pinch of salt

Preheat the oven to 180°C, 350°F, Gas mark 4.

Drain the beans that have been soaking overnight and put them in a saucepan. Cover with water and bring to the boil. Cook, uncovered, for 30 minutes in boiling water, then drain well in a colander. Don't worry that the beans are not tender – they are meant to be half cooked.

Meanwhile, make the rose harissa: put the red (bell) pepper, onion and garlic on a baking tray and drizzle with olive oil. Roast in the preheated oven for about 30 minutes or so, until cooked and tender. Set aside to cool and then cut the red (bell) pepper in half, remove the stalk, ribs and seeds, and peel off the blistered skin. Peel the garlic cloves, squeezing out the garlic inside.

Blend all the rose harissa ingredients, including the roasted vegetables, to a smooth paste in a food processor.

Preheat the oven to 150°C, 300°F, Gas mark 2. Score the boned shoulder of lamb in a criss-cross pattern and then rub half the rose harissa mixture into the lamb.

Put the semi-cooked beans, sliced red onion, thyme and chicken broth in an ovenproof casserole dish. Lay the lamb on top and bake in the preheated oven for 3½ hours.

When cooked, lift out the lamb and place it on a carving board. Skim off any excess fat from the top of the beans, then stir in the remaining rose harissa paste. Check the seasoning, adding some salt and pepper if required.

Carve the lamb into slices and serve with the warm beans.

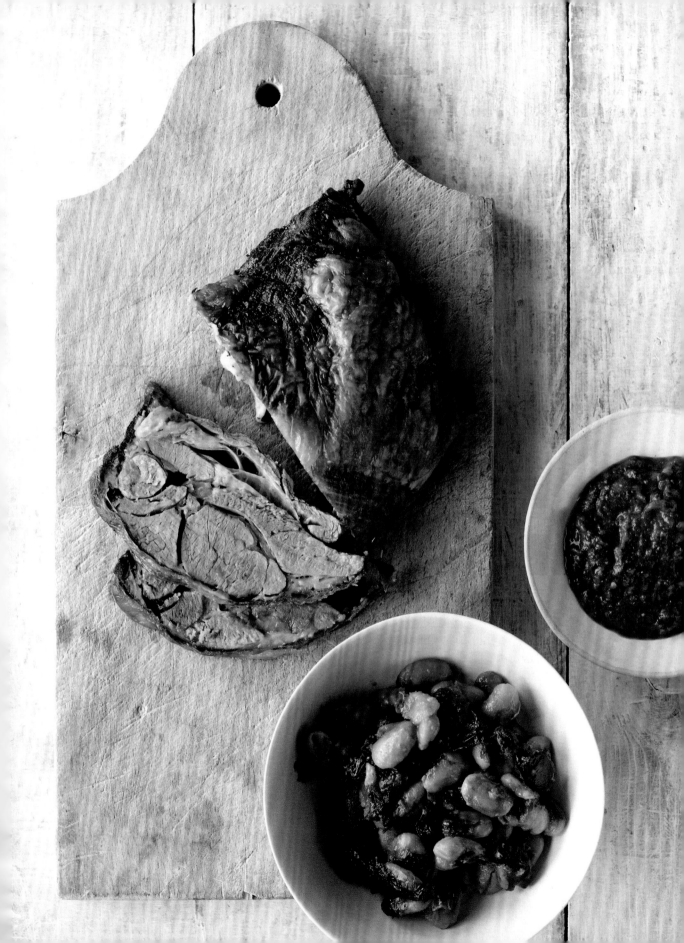

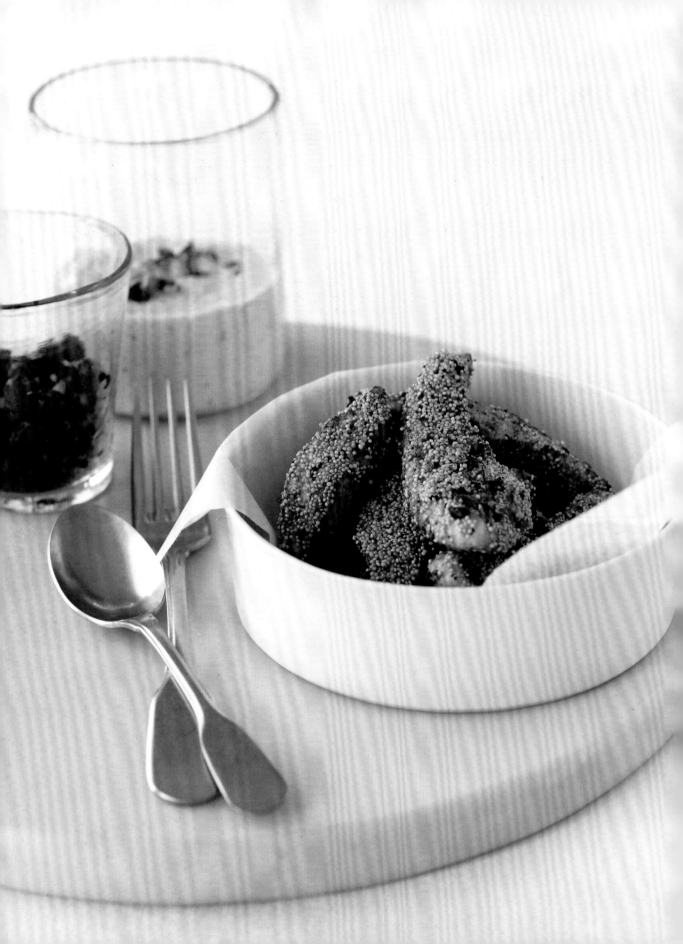

P+ Amaranth chicken strips with pomegranate & fig yoghurt

Amaranth is a brilliant gluten-free grain, which crisps beautifully when used as a coating for poultry and fish. The ras-el-hanout adds depth of flavour and the yoghurt sauce lends natural sweetness. You can make this the day before and serve cold with a blanched salad.

Serves 4

400g (14oz) chicken breast, cut into fine strips

20g (¾oz) coconut oil

few pomegranate seeds to garnish

For the coating:

pinch of finely ground sea salt

40g (1½oz) amaranth, cooked in a dry hot pan for 30 seconds until it pops

2 tsp ras-el-hanout

80g (3oz) coconut oil

For the pomegranate & fig yoghurt:

150ml (5fl oz/scant ⅔ cup) pomegranate juice

80ml (3fl oz/scant ⅓ cup) orange juice

40g (1½oz) dried figs, finely sliced

pinch of ras-el-hanout

few mint sprigs, chopped

few coriander (cilantro) sprigs, chopped

40ml (1½fl oz/3 tbsp) 24-hour fermented yoghurt (see page 52)

Mix all the ingredients for the coating in a large bowl and then use to coat each piece of chicken, shaking off the excess coating. Cover and place in the fridge until ready to cook.

To make the pomegranate and fig yoghurt, pour the pomegranate juice and orange juice into a small pan. Add the sliced figs and bring to the boil. Cook over a medium heat until the liquid has reduced almost completely. Remove from the heat and set aside to cool. When cool, mix together the fig syrup, ras-el-hanout, chopped mint and coriander (cilantro) and the yoghurt.

Shallow-fry the chicken strips in the coconut oil over a medium heat for about 2 minutes on each side until golden brown and cooked right through.

Serve the chicken immediately with a large spoonful of yoghurt and a sprinkling of pomegranate seeds.

NUTRITION FACTS

Amaranth dates back to pre-Colombian times and was used by the Aztecs. It is rich in calcium, magnesium and iron, which are all required for energy and heart health, with vitamin B6 for healing and repair.

(P+) Crisp lentil-coated crayfish cakes with coconut & mango

This takes fishcakes to a whole new level. The Asian flavours are unmistakable, ensuring that the cakes stay fresh and crisp. Lentils and black sesame seeds provide a superb coating, which is neither glutinous nor sweet – make double the quantity to store in the fridge.

Serves 4

100g (3½oz) cooked crayfish tails, drained and squeezed dry

100g (3½oz) white fish (e.g. cod, pollock or haddock), skinned and boned

10g (½oz) fresh root ginger, finely diced

1 lemongrass stalk, peeled and finely chopped

2 spring onions (scallions), finely chopped

1 fresh red chilli, deseeded and chopped

20g (¾oz) coriander (cilantro), stalks only, finely chopped

grated zest of ½ lime

2 tsp Thai fish sauce (nam pla)

30g (1¼oz) coconut oil for frying

50g (2oz/⅓ cup) split red lentils, ground in a spice grinder to flour

pinch of black sesame seeds

For the coconut sauce:

200ml (7fl oz/generous ¾ cup) coconut milk

½ fresh red chilli, chopped

20g (¾oz) fresh root ginger, peeled and grated

50ml (2fl oz/scant ¼ cup) lime juice

1 tsp local runny honey

20ml (4 tsp) Thai fish sauce (nam pla)

For the mango salad:

40g (1½oz) fresh mango, peeled, stoned and cut into 1cm (½in) dice

few coriander (cilantro) sprigs, finely chopped

few mint sprigs, finely chopped

2 spring onions (scallions), thinly sliced

1 tsp lime juice

2 tsp olive oil

To make the fishcakes, finely chop the crayfish and white fish together, so that they start to stick to each other. In a large mixing bowl, mix the chopped fish with the ginger, lemongrass, spring onions (scallions), chilli, chopped coriander (cilantro), lime zest and fish sauce. Divide the mixture into 8 portions and shape each one into a small patty. Cover and keep in the fridge until ready to cook.

Make the coconut sauce: put all the ingredients in a small thick-based saucepan and reduce by boiling vigorously over a high heat by two-thirds. Set aside and keep warm.

Meanwhile, make the mango salad by mixing all the ingredients together in a small bowl.

When you're ready to cook the fishcakes, heat a small frying pan over a medium heat and melt the coconut oil. Mix together the lentil flour and sesame seeds and use to lightly coat the fishcakes. Fry for 2 minutes on each side until golden brown.

Drain the fishcakes on kitchen paper and serve with the coconut sauce and mango salad.

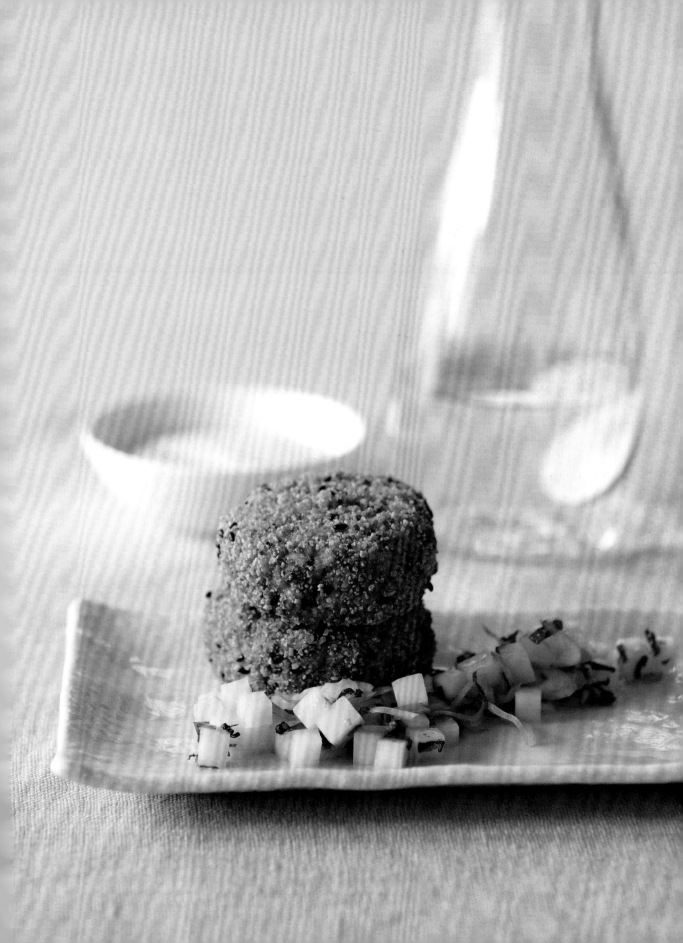

(P+) Confit of salmon with bulghur salad & tapenade

This is restaurant-level cuisine, suitable for dinner parties, but easier to make than it looks. Prepare the tapenade and salad separately and store in the fridge overnight. Cook the salmon on the day of eating. You can eat it cold for lunch with a blanched salad.

Serves 4

8g (⅓oz) salt

1 tbsp local runny honey

200ml (7fl oz/generous ¾ cup) warm water

300g (10oz) salmon fillet

Walnut, tarragon, shallot & honey dressing (see page 212)

For the tapenade:

200g (7oz/1½ cups) black olives (Niçoise or Kalamata), pitted

1 garlic clove

80ml (3fl oz/scant ⅓ cup) olive oil

50g (2oz/¼ cup) capers

20g (¾oz) fresh parsley

20g (¾oz) anchovy fillets

4 tsp lemon juice

ground black pepper

50g (2oz/generous ½ cup) roasted walnuts

1 tbsp Dijon mustard

For the bulghur salad:

20g (¾oz) bulghur wheat

10g (½oz) red quinoa

few parsley sprigs, chopped

few mint sprigs, chopped

1 tbsp olive oil

1 tsp lemon juice

2 large tomatoes, skinned, deseeded and cut into fine dice

To make the confit salmon, mix the salt, honey and warm water together in a bowl. Stir to dissolve the salt and set aside to cool. Immerse the salmon fillet in this liquid and leave it submerged in the fridge for 1 hour.

Remove from the fridge and place the salmon on a long piece of cling film (plastic wrap) on a board. Using the cling film (plastic wrap), roll the salmon into a sausage shape. Twist the ends tightly to seal it and then roll in another layer of cling film (plastic wrap).

Place the salmon in a large saucepan and cover it with cold water. Put a smaller lid inside the pan to push the salmon under the water. Over a high heat, bring the water to a gentle boil, then remove from the heat and allow the water to cool with the salmon still submerged. When cold, remove the salmon from the pan, still wrapped in cling film (plastic wrap), and refrigerate.

Make the tapenade: blend all the ingredients together in a food processor until smooth. Keep in an airtight container in the fridge.

Make the bulghur salad: cook the bulghur wheat and quinoa in a saucepan of boiling water for 20 minutes. Then refresh under cold running water and drain. In a small bowl, mix the cooked grains with the other ingredients.

Cut the salmon, still wrapped in the cling film (plastic wrap), into 4 slices and then remove the cling film (plastic wrap). Serve the salmon on top of the bulghur salad with the tapenade and drizzle some of the dressing around it.

CHEF'S TIP

The secret is to roll and wrap the salmon as tightly as possible, and only remove the cling film (plastic wrap) once it has cooled and 'set' to prevent it unravelling.

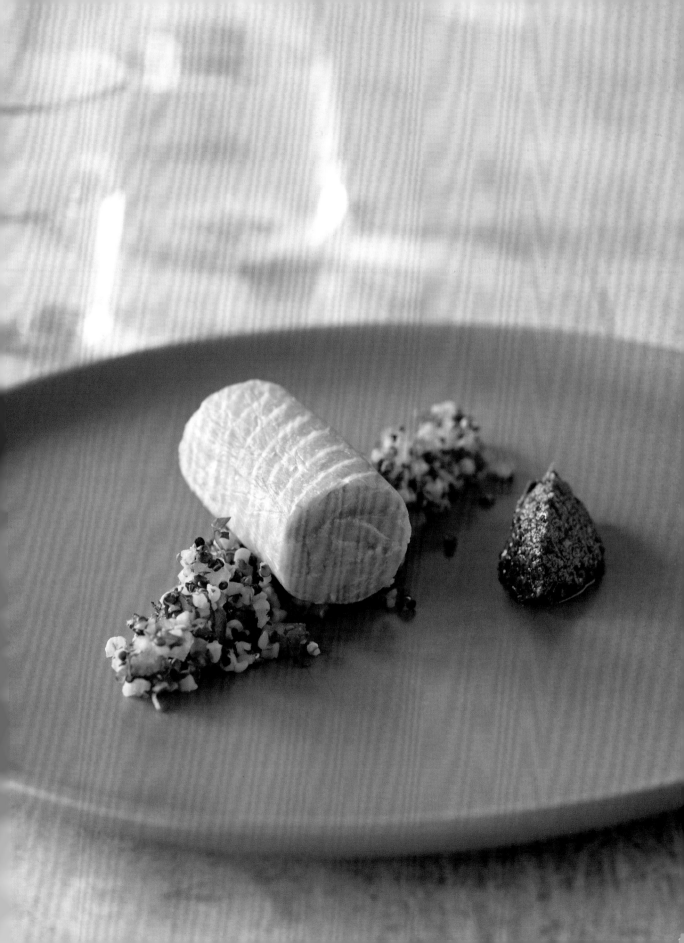

(P+) Butter bean hummus with salsa & quinoa flatbreads

If you don't want to eat meat, poultry and fish all the time, this vegetarian option is really easy to assemble and packed with vegetable proteins. You can make a larger quantity of hummus to store in the fridge, if wished. The delicious quinoa flatbreads contain essential fats and protein.

Serves 6

175g (6oz/1 cup) dried butter (lima) beans (soaked in cold water overnight with a squeeze of lemon juice)

2 tbsp lemon juice

large pinch of salt

grated zest of ½ lemon

1 tbsp tahini

3 tbsp extra virgin olive oil

1 garlic clove, thinly sliced

1 tsp ground cumin

1 tsp ground coriander

20g (¾oz) coriander (cilantro)

50ml (2fl oz/scant ¼ cup) cold water

Avocado, chipotle & tomato salsa (see page 77)

small bunch of pea shoots

For the quinoa flatbreads:

100g (3½oz/¾ cup) quinoa flour, plus extra for dusting

50g (2oz) shelled hemp

pinch of salt

½ tsp paprika

1 tsp olive oil

a little warm water to mix

Drain the soaked beans and place them in a saucepan. Cover them with fresh cold water and bring slowly to the boil, then reduce the heat and simmer gently for about 50 minutes until the beans are tender and cooked. Drain in a colander and set aside.

In a small bowl, mix together the lemon juice, salt, lemon zest and tahini.

In a small frying pan, warm the oil, garlic, cumin and ground coriander together over a low heat until the garlic is golden brown. Remove from the heat and add the lemon juice mixture immediately to stop the garlic overcooking. (Take care not to burn the garlic or it will be very bitter.)

Place the cooked beans in a blender jug with the oil and garlic mixture and fresh coriander (cilantro). Blend to a smooth paste, adding enough water to achieve a thick dipping consistency. Keep in a sealed container in the fridge for up to 4 days.

To make the flatbreads, mix together the quinoa flour, hemp, salt and paprika in a large bowl. Mix the olive oil with the warm water and slowly add to the mixture to make a dough. Turn it out on to a lightly floured work surface (use some quinoa flour) and knead lightly. Divide the dough into 8 pieces and then roll each one into an oval or round. Layer with greaseproof paper on a plate, then cover with cling film (plastic wrap) and leave in the fridge until ready to cook.

To cook the flatbreads, heat a large frying pan over a medium heat and dry-fry them for 1 minute on each side.

Serve the warm flatbreads with the hummus, the Avocado, chipotle and tomato salsa and some pea shoots.

VARIATION

You can change the flavour of the hummus by adding fresh basil or mint instead of coriander (cilantro).

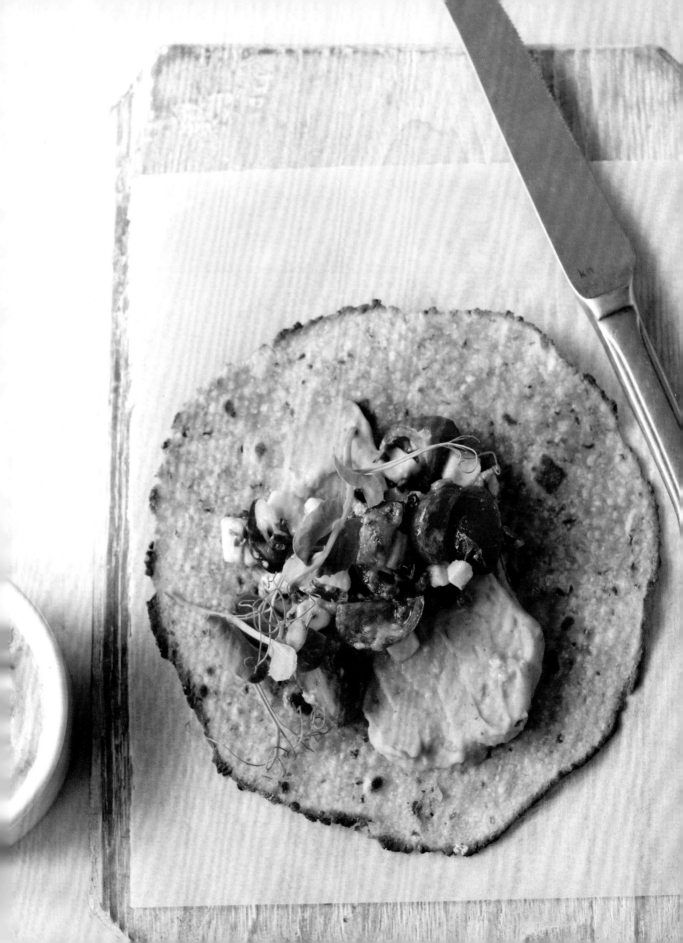

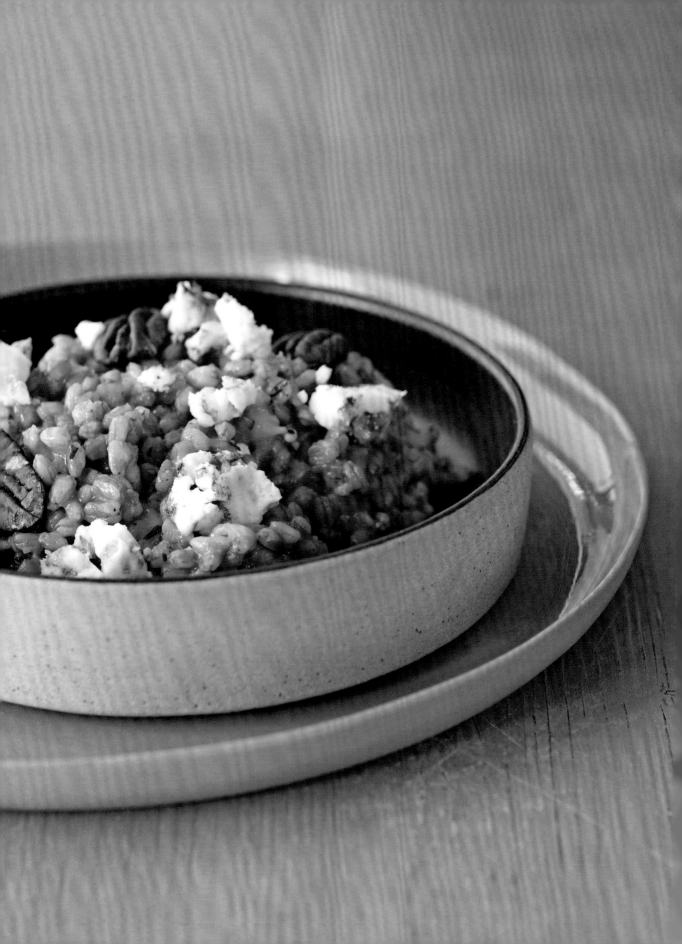

P+ Spelt risotto with celeriac, spinach & roquefort

Spelt has a wonderful nutty texture, which lends itself to risotto, whilst the spinach and melting Roquefort enhance the flavour. Use goat's cheese instead if cow's dairy is off your Allowed Foods list. Serve this risotto hot or cold with a blanched salad for a take-to-work lunch.

Serves 4

20g (¾oz/1½ tbsp) unsalted butter

40g (1½oz) shallots, chopped

200g (7oz) celeriac, peeled and cut into 2cm (1in) chunks

few thyme sprigs, stalks removed and leaves finely chopped

250g (8oz) spelt, soaked in boiling water for 10 minutes and then drained

75ml (3fl oz/5 tbsp) dry white wine

1 litre (1¾ pints/4 cups) hot Chicken Broth (see page 44)

40g (1½oz/½ cup) pecans, halved

100g (3½oz) baby spinach leaves, washed

100g (3½oz) Roquefort, cut into 1cm (½in) dice

ground black pepper

Heat a large thick-based pan over a medium heat. Melt the butter and sauté the shallots, celeriac and thyme until the shallots are soft with no colour. Add the drained spelt and white wine and cook until the wine has reduced by two-thirds.

Add a couple of ladles of hot chicken broth to the pan and, using a wooden spoon, stir over a medium heat until most of the liquid has been absorbed by the spelt. Continue to add the broth, little by little, bringing it back to the boil whilst stirring and shaking the pan. Every 45 seconds, add some more broth until the spelt is cooked through. There's no need to stir the risotto as frequently towards the end. The whole process will take about 20 minutes.

Meanwhile, roast the pecans in a preheated oven at 170°C, 325°F, Gas mark 3 for 8 minutes.

When the risotto is cooked, remove from the heat and add the spinach and Roquefort. The spinach will wilt and the Roquefort will melt into the risotto. Season to taste with black pepper and serve in warmed bowls with a sprinkling of roasted pecans.

NUTRITION FACTS

Spelt is an ancient grain which is related to the wheat family, but it is far lower in gluten as well as being higher in Omega-3 and -6 for a healthy heart.

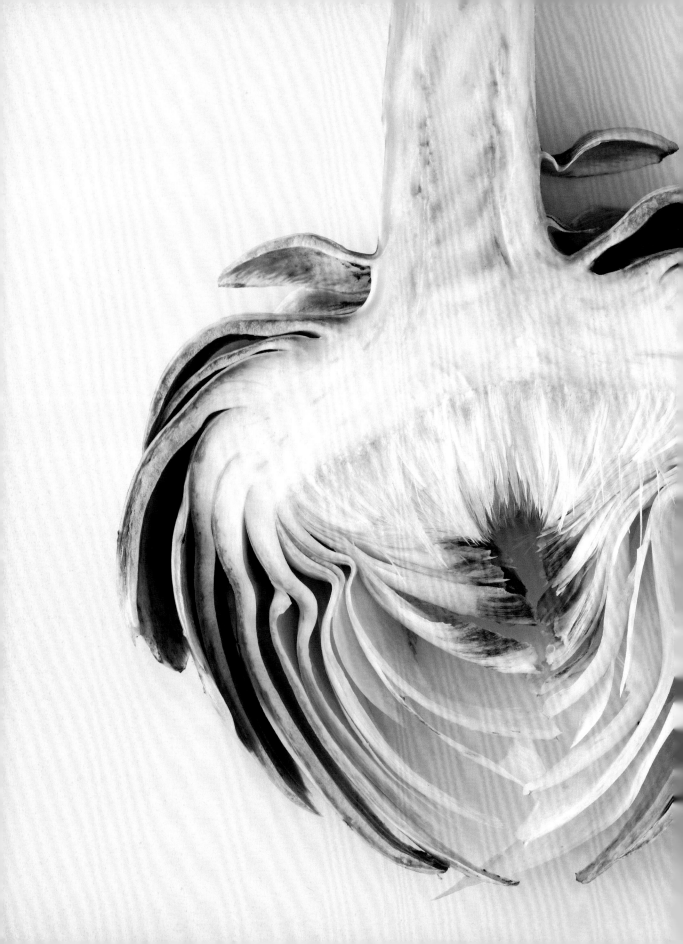

Vegetable side dishes

(P) Jerk-spiced roast butternut squash with citrus salsa

Butternut squash is the perfect substitute for the usual accompaniment of potatoes, rice and other grains as it is has a sweet flavour and can be mashed on the plate. Packed with beta-carotene and vitamin C to boost your immunity, this delicious dish is irresistible.

Serves 4

500g (1lb 2oz) butternut squash

For the jerk marinade:

1 tsp ground cinnamon

2 tsp ground coriander

½ tsp ground black pepper

1 tsp ground allspice

1 tsp freshly grated nutmeg

pinch of salt

2 tbsp thyme leaves stripped from the stalks

15g (½oz) fresh root ginger, peeled and grated

½ small Scotch bonnet chilli, deseeded

juice of 1 lime

6 spring onions (scallions)

30g (1oz/2 tbsp) clarified butter

2 garlic cloves

For the mango salsa:

1 lemon, segmented and juice reserved

2 oranges, segmented and juice reserved

250g (8oz) ripe mango, peeled, stoned and cut into 5mm (¼in) dice

few coriander (cilantro) sprigs, chopped

pinch of sea salt

4 red spring onions (scallions), chopped

½ Scotch bonnet chilli, deseeded and finely chopped

pinch of ground allspice

4 tsp olive oil

Preheat the oven to 200°C, 400°F, Gas mark 6.

Peel the butternut squash, using a potato peeler, and remove the seeds with a dessertspoon. Cut it into discs, about 1cm (¼in) thick.

Blend all the ingredients for the jerk marinade in a food processor until the mixture forms a thick paste. You might need to add a dash of cold water to loosen it a little.

Mix the butternut squash into the marinade and then place on a parchment-lined baking sheet ready for cooking later.

Make the salsa: chop the citrus fruit segments into 5mm (¼in) chunks. In a stainless steel bowl, mix all the ingredients together and set aside for at least 1 hour. The salsa is best made the day before and kept in the fridge overnight (it will keep for 5 days).

Roast the jerk-spiced butternut squash in the preheated oven for about 20–25 minutes, turning occasionally, until the edges are just starting to char slightly.

Remove from the oven and serve the warm squash, drizzled with the salsa. If wished, this can be eaten cold as a salad.

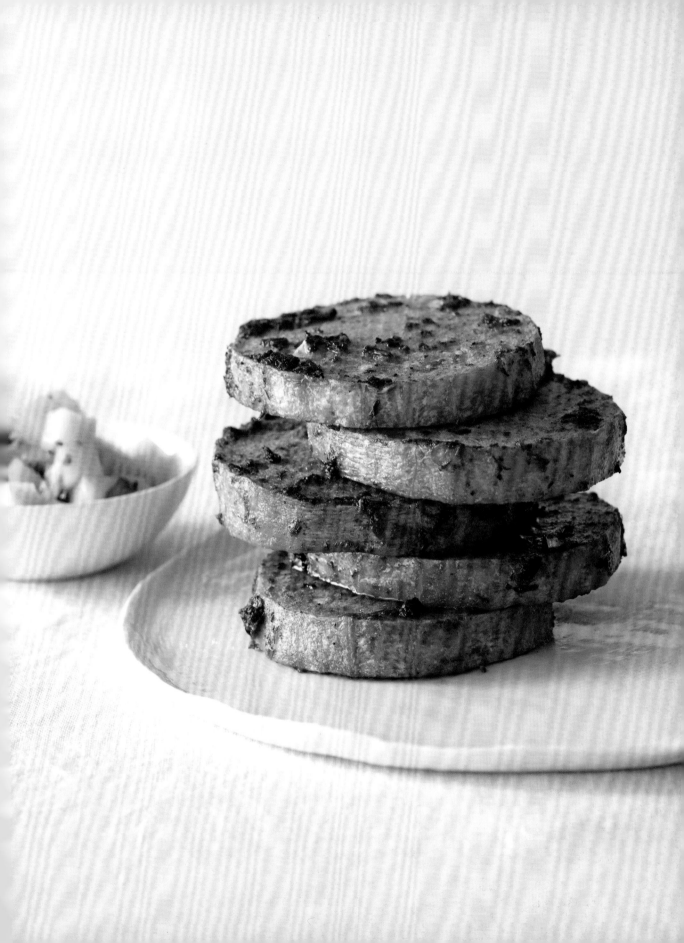

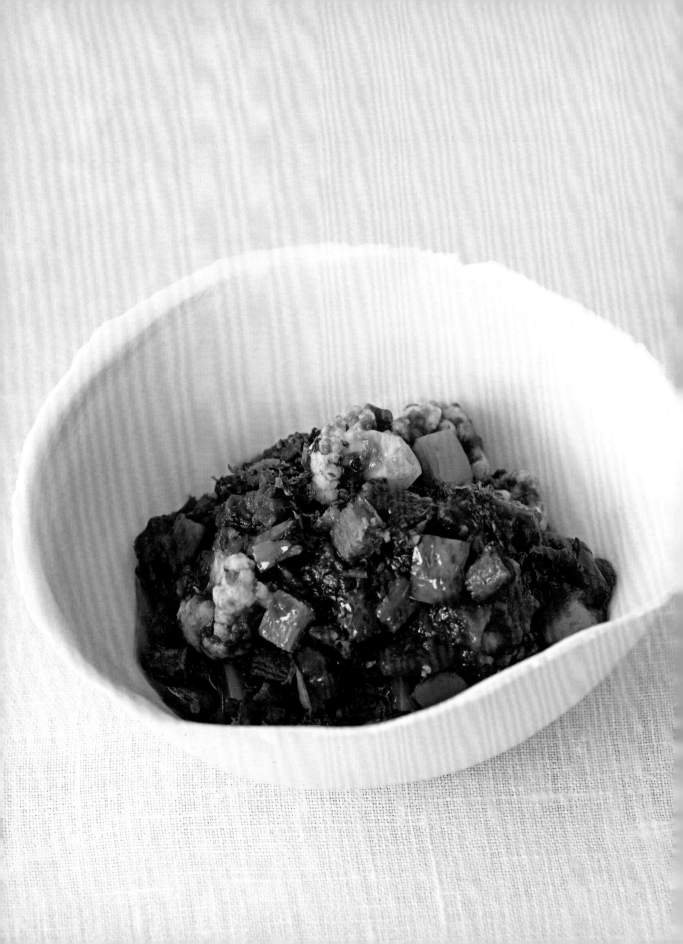

Ⓟ Roasted cauliflower ratatouille

When cauliflower cheese is out of the question, combining cauliflower with ratatouille brings both parts of the dish alive. The marriage of Mediterranean vegetables and traditional herbs is heightened with the nutmeg, allspice and apple cider vinegar – mouthwatering!

Serves 6

150g (5oz) cauliflower florets

80g (3oz) red (bell) pepper, deseeded and cut into 1cm (½in) chunks

80g (3oz) yellow (bell) pepper, deseeded and cut into 1cm (½in) chunks

80g (3oz) green (bell) pepper, deseeded and cut into 1cm (½in) chunks

50g (2oz) red onion, thinly sliced

50g (2oz) courgette (zucchini), cut into 1cm (½in) chunks

olive oil for drizzling

1 tbsp chopped rosemary leaves

1 tbsp chopped thyme leaves

sea salt and ground black pepper

For the sauce:

10g (½oz) coconut oil

1 small onion, finely chopped

3 garlic cloves, crushed

1 cinnamon stick

2 bay leaves

2 thyme sprigs

2 allspice berries, finely crushed

1 tsp local runny honey

2 tsp cider vinegar

150ml (¼ pint/scant ⅔ cup) Chicken Broth (see page 44)

200g (7oz) canned chopped tomatoes

chopped flat-leaf parsley to garnish

Preheat the oven to 200°C, 400°F, Gas mark 6.

Blanch the cauliflower in a pan of boiling water for 1 minute, then drain and refresh in cold water. Pat dry with kitchen paper.

Put the (bell) peppers, red onion, cauliflower florets and courgette (zucchini) on a non-stick baking tray and drizzle with the oil. Add the chopped herbs and season with salt and pepper. Roast in the preheated oven for 15–20 minutes until golden brown, turning the vegetables halfway though cooking. Remove and keep warm.

Make the sauce: in a thick-based pan, melt the coconut oil over a medium heat and gently sweat the onion and garlic with the cinnamon, bay leaves, thyme and allspice until golden brown, stirring continuously.

Add the honey, cider vinegar, chicken broth and chopped tomatoes. Reduce the heat to a gentle simmer and cook for 20 minutes. Season to taste with salt and pepper and remove the cinnamon, bay leaves and thyme before adding the roasted vegetables. Cook for 5 minutes to bring all the flavours together.

Serve the ratatouille warm with lots of chopped parsley.

P Pak choi with lentils & lime

Anyone who considers lentils bland should try this spicy combination. You can prepare the lentils the day before, if wished, adding the freshly cooked pak choi just before serving. The secret is to taste the lime juice through the coconut milk in order to attain the right balance.

Serves 4

50g (2oz/scant ⅓ cup) Puy lentils, soaked overnight with a squeeze of lemon juice, then boiled in water for 20 minutes

50g (2oz/¼ cup) red lentils, soaked in boiling water with a squeeze of lemon juice

50g (2oz/scant ⅓ cup) green lentils, soaked overnight with a dash of lemon juice, then boiled in water for 20 minutes

8 large pak choi

fresh lime and coriander (cilantro) to garnish

For the curry sauce:

150g (5oz) onion, sliced

20g (¾oz) garlic, crushed

50g (2oz) carrot, finely chopped

20g (¾oz) coconut oil

30g (1oz/scant ¼ cup) dried unsulphured apricots, chopped

1 tsp cumin seeds

1 tsp coriander seeds

1 tsp fennel seeds

½ tsp ground turmeric

10g (½oz) roasted garam masala

5 green cardamom pods, bashed in half with a pestle and mortar

2 fresh red chillies, deseeded and finely chopped

8g (⅓oz) fresh root ginger, peeled and grated

5 tomatoes, cut into quarters

200ml (7fl oz/generous ¾ cup) coconut milk

3 tbsp lime juice

finely grated zest of 1 lime

3 tbsp chopped coriander (cilantro)

pinch of salt

To make the curry sauce, sweat the onion, garlic and carrot in the coconut oil over a low heat until soft and golden brown. Add the apricots, spices, chilli and ginger and cook for 2 minutes, stirring continuously. Add the tomatoes, coconut milk and a dash of water. Cover the pan and cook gently for 20 minutes, stirring occasionally.

Remove from the heat, add the lime juice and zest, coriander (cilantro) and salt and blitz in a jug blender until it's smooth. Pass the sauce through a fine sieve into a clean pan.

Add the cooked lentils to the sauce and warm through gently. Check that you can taste the lime cutting through the richness of the coconut (you may need to add a little more lime juice).

To prepare the pak choi, cut it in half lengthways and blanch in a pan of boiling salted water for 1 minute, then drain well. Pour the lentil curry into serving bowls and top with the pak choi. Serve garnished with fresh lime and coriander (cilantro).

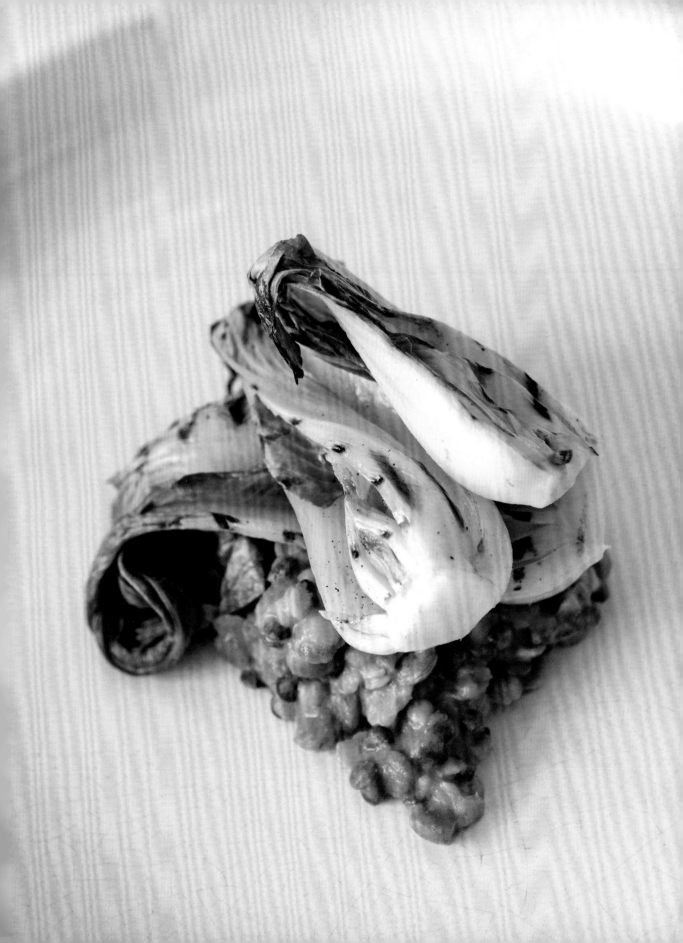

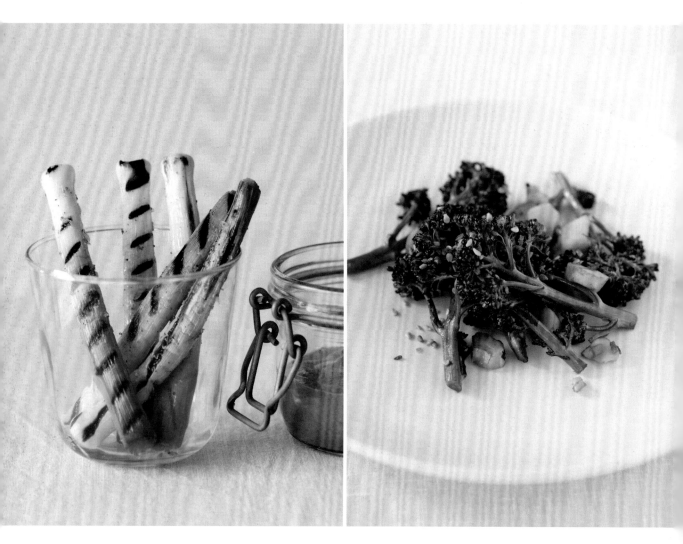

Grilled baby leeks with romesco sauce

Purple sprouting broccoli with brazil nuts, sesame & orange

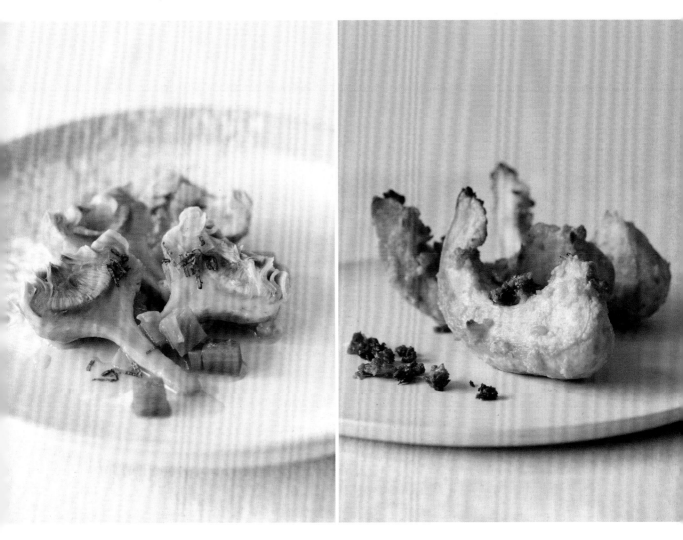

Artichoke barigoule

Roasted pumpkin with chilli, cashews & lemon

(P) Grilled baby leeks with romesco sauce

Romesco sauce is a delicous way of eating peppers and is great served with leeks. A mixture of almonds and hazelnuts are combined with sherry vinegar, sweet paprika and piquillo peppers to add fire to the gentle flavour of the leeks, while providing you with protein and essential fats.

Serves 4

24 baby leeks, trimmed

20g (¾oz) clarified butter, melted

salt and black pepper, to taste

For the romesco sauce:

30g (1oz/scant ⅓ cup) whole shelled almonds,

30g (1oz/scant ⅓ cup) whole shelled hazelnuts

2 tbsp extra virgin olive oil

1 garlic clove, thinly sliced

4 tsp lemon juice

150g (5oz) piquillo peppers (or roasted red (bell) pepper)

1 tsp smoked sweet paprika

2 tsp sherry vinegar

pinch of sea salt

Preheat the oven to 170°C, 325°F, Gas mark 3.

Bring a large pan of salted water to the boil and blanch the leeks for 1 minute. Drain well and arrange the leeks on a plate. Drizzle the warm clarified butter over the top, and season with salt and pepper ready for grilling later.

Make the romesco sauce: put the almonds and hazelnuts on a non-stick baking tray and roast in the preheated oven for 20 minutes. Rub the nuts in a clean tea towel to remove the skins.

In a small pan, gently heat the olive oil over a low heat and fry the garlic until golden brown. Remove from the heat and add the lemon juice (this will stop the garlic over-colouring and becoming bitter).

In a food processor, blend the garlic and nuts with all the other sauce ingredients, using the pulse button. You might need to add a little water if the romesco is too thick. (I like it quite chunky in texture rather than smooth – it is less dry.) The romesco will keep in a sealed container in the fridge for up to 1 week.

Heat a griddle pan over a high heat and grill the leeks for 2 minutes on each side until they are charred and ready to dip into the romesco.

VARIATION

Alternatively, you can grill the leeks over hot coals on a barbecue for a really smoky flavour.

(P) Purple sprouting broccoli with brazil nuts, sesame & orange

This vegetable dish is really quick and easy to make, and the combination of orange, tamari and sesame is divine. The layering of flavours here is key to the dish's success, but always make sure that you fry nuts and seeds at a low temperature to prevent them from browning and turning the fats rancid.

Serves 4

200g (7oz) purple sprouting broccoli

10g (½oz/1 tbsp) clarified butter

40g (1½oz/scant ½ cup) Brazil nuts, finely sliced

10g (½oz) white sesame seeds

1 garlic clove, crushed

4 tsp Tamari

grated zest of ½ orange

2 tsp sesame oil

Bring a pan of salted water to the boil and blanch the broccoli for 3½ minutes. Drain well in a colander.

Place a wok over a low heat, add the butter and fry the Brazil nuts for 1 minute. Add the sesame seeds and cook for approximately 1 minute until they start to pop. Increase the heat, then add the garlic and cook for 30 seconds. Stir in the blanched broccoli.

Stir-fry for 1–2 minutes before adding the Tamari, orange zest and sesame oil.

Serve immediately on a warmed dish.

(P) Artichoke barigoule

This is a grown-up version of a simple but highly nutritious supper. Artichokes are great for the digestion, liver, gall bladder and kidneys as they act as a natural diuretic. They also help to stave off food cravings, making this so much more than just another vegetable dish.

Serves 4

12 violet baby artichokes

juice of 1 lemon

1 litre (1¾ pints/4 cups) water

30g (1oz/2 tbsp) clarified butter

100g (3½oz) carrot, cut into 2mm (⅛in) dice

100g (3½oz) shallot, cut into 2mm (⅛in) dice

80g (3oz) celery, cut into 2mm (⅛in) dice

1 garlic clove, diced

250ml (8fl oz/1 cup) dry white wine

1 tsp chopped tarragon

750ml (1¼ pints/3 cups) Chicken Broth (see page 44)

Place the artichokes on a chopping board and trim them to the top two-thirds just above the choke. Add the lemon juice to the water in a large bowl and dip the trimmed artichokes into this acidulated water to prevent it browning. Place the artichokes on the board, choke-side down, and snap off the tough outer leaves to just expose the outer part of the choke.Keep the trimmed artichokes in the bowl of acidulated water until you are ready to cook them.

In a large pan, melt the butter over a medium heat and sauté the carrot, shallot, celery and garlic for about 5 minutes until the shallot and garlic soften and have no colour. Add the drained prepared artichokes and cook for 2 minutes before adding the white wine.

Cook rapidly to reduce by one-half, then add the tarragon and chicken broth. Simmer, covered with a lid, over a gentle heat for 15 minutes. Remove the pan from the heat and leave the artichokes in the cooking liquid. They will go on cooking as the liquid cools.

Serve the artichokes either hot or cold with a little Walnut, tarragon, shallot & honey dressing (see page 212).

(P) Roasted pumpkin with chilli, cashews & lemon

The clumps of spiced cashews, chilli and lemon cling to the orange flesh of the pumpkin, which caramelizes when it is roasted. Adding a subtle Asian flavouring to a traditional English root vegetable with its sprinkle of black onion seeds is an unexpected yet delightful twist.

Serves 4

900g (2lb) pumpkin

125g (4oz/scant 1 cup) cashew nuts

10g (½oz) fresh green chilli

1 garlic clove

1 tbsp local runny honey

finely grated zest and juice of 1 lemon plus extra for squeezing

80ml (3fl oz/scant ⅓ cup) water

1 tbsp roasted garam masala

1 tsp black onion seeds plus extra for sprinkling

Preheat the oven to 200°C, 400°F, Gas mark 6.

Peel and deseed the pumpkin. Slice the flesh into 1cm (½in) thick rounds or wedges. In a food processor, blitz all the other ingredients to a paste.

Line a large roasting tray with a silicone non-stick sheet or silicone paper.

In a large bowl, coat the pumpkin all over with the cashew paste and then arrange on the roasting tray. Roast in the preheated oven for about 30 minutes until tender and golden brown.

Serve warm with a sprinkle of black onion seeds and a squeeze of lemon.

Ⓟ Salt-baked celeriac

Celeriac is one of the most under-used vegetables, and yet it is deliciously sweet when baked in a salt crust, as all the moisture and nutrients are held inside when it's cooked in this way. Because only the centre of the celeriac is eaten, you will not consume any flour in the crust.

Serves 4–6

300g (10oz) sea salt crystals

400g (13oz/3⅓ cups) plain (all-purpose) flour

20g (¾oz) rosemary leaves, chopped

250ml (8fl oz/1 cup) cold water

1kg (2lb 3½oz) celeriac, thoroughly washed and trimmed

Preheat the oven to 170°C, 325°F, Gas mark 3.

In a large mixing bowl, mix the salt, flour and rosemary together. Pour in the cold water and bring together with your hands to form a thick dough.

On a lightly floured board, roll out the dough to 5mm (¼in) thick – it should be large enough to encase the celeriac. Place the celeriac on the dough and cover it, sealing the top by pushing together the edges of the dough to form a tight seal. Place on a non-stick baking sheet.

Bake in the preheated oven for 2½–3 hours. Remove and then crack the top-third of the crust with a serrated small knife.

Serve whole in a dish with a spoon to scoop out the celeriac.

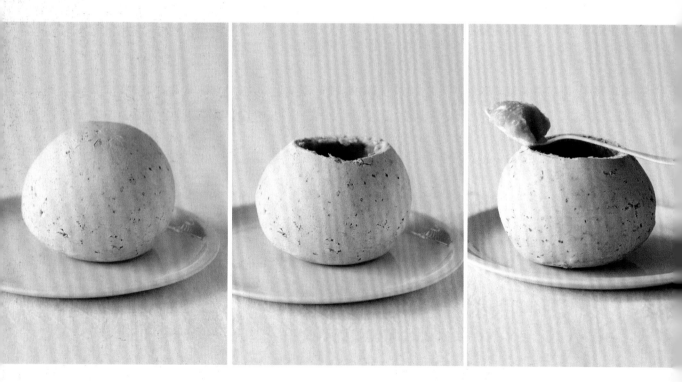

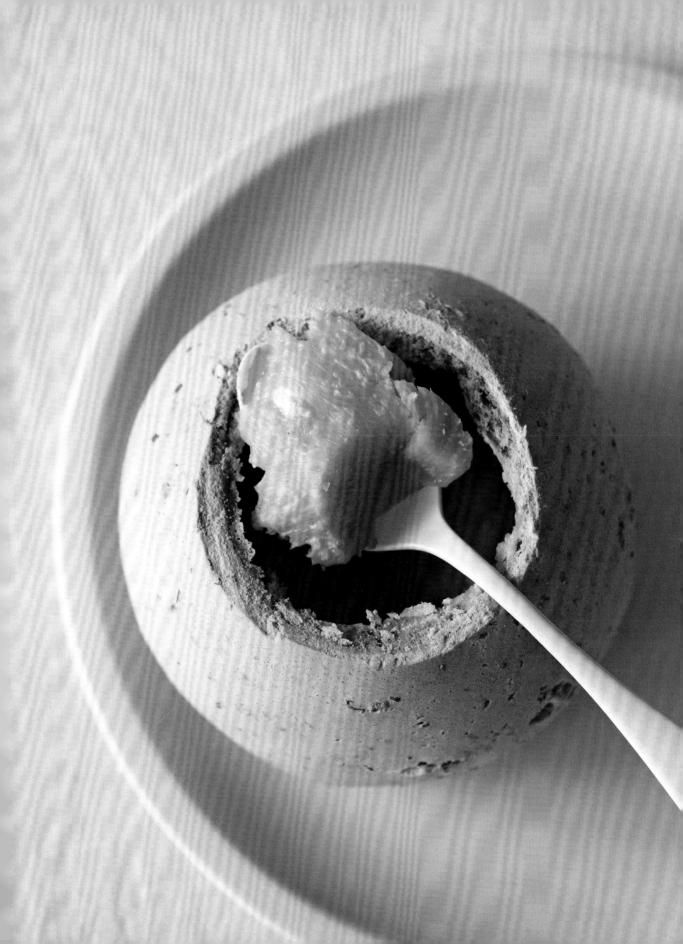

(P) Green beans with hazelnut & pea pesto

It is often the combination of colour, taste and texture that really makes a dish, as is shown by this method of serving green beans. The creaminess of the pea and hazelnut pesto, the moisture and freshness of the beans, and the crunch of the toasted hazelnuts complement each other perfectly.

Serves 4

350g (12oz) fine green beans, trimmed

20g (¾oz/⅛ cup) roasted hazelnuts, skins removed

For the hazelnut & pea pesto:

300g (10oz/2½ cups) frozen peas, blanched in boiling water and refreshed

1 tbsp chopped mint

50g (2oz/¼ cup) roasted hazelnuts, skins removed

1 small garlic clove

ground black pepper

pinch of salt

100ml (3½fl oz/generous ⅓ cup) extra virgin olive oil

Make the pesto: using a pestle and mortar, grind all the ingredients together, except the olive oil, until smooth. Then gradually stir in the olive oil. Keep covered in the fridge for up to 4 days.

Blanch the green beans in a pan of boiling water for 2–3 minutes. Drain in a colander.

Serve the beans in a warmed dish with a few dollops of the pea pesto and a scattering of roasted hazelnuts.

P Roasted beetroot with chipotle, tangerine & pistachios

Beetroot (beets) takes on a more meaty flavour when it is roasted rather than simply boiled or simmered, and this cooking method also preserves far more of its nutrients. The tangerines contribute some additional antioxidants, making this Middle Eastern-style dish an overall immune-booster.

Serves 4

20g (¾oz) coconut oil

2 tangerines, juiced and zested

850g (1lb 13oz) raw beetroots (beets), mixed colours, peeled, sliced and diced

1 tbsp chopped pistachios

1 tsp Tangerine, cumin, fennel & chipotle salt (see page 36)

Preheat the oven to 180°C, 350°F, Gas mark 4. Line a large baking sheet with some greaseproof paper.

Gently warm the coconut oil in a small pan until melted. Remove from the heat.

In a large bowl, mix together the warmed coconut oil and the tangerine juice and zest. Stir in the diced beetroot (beets) and when it's well coated pour onto the lined baking sheet.

Roast in the preheated oven for approximately 50 minutes until the beetroot (beets) is cooked and tender – turn it once or twice during cooking.

To serve, transfer the beetroot (beets) to a dish and sprinkle with the chopped pistachios. Season with the Tangerine, cumin, fennel and chipotle salt.

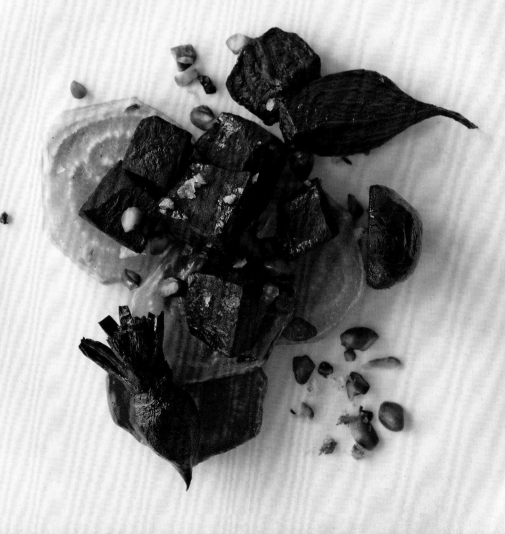

Ⓟ Slow-roasted peppers, aubergines, anchovies & almonds

Aubergine (eggplant) is not chosen very often as many of us don't know how best to cook it. Baking in foil in the oven brings out its natural smoky taste and when it's combined with the strongly flavoured anchovies, this vegetable comes alive in a marvelous dish that you will want to repeat.

Serves 4

2 large aubergines (eggplants)
2 red (bell) peppers
1 medium onion, unpeeled
4 tsp olive oil
10g (½oz) flat-leaf parsley
4 tsp sherry vinegar
pinch of salt
8 anchovy fillets
40g (1½oz/¼ cup) whole roasted almonds
1 tsp sweet smoked paprika

Preheat the oven to 180°C, 350°F, Gas mark 4.

Wrap the aubergines (eggplants), peppers and onion in kitchen foil and roast in the preheated oven for 1½ hours.

Remove from the oven and allow the vegetables to cool slightly. Remove the skin from the onion and cut into 8 wedges, reserving a few pieces as a garnish. Remove the skins, seeds and stalks from the peppers and shred the flesh finely. Remove the skin from the aubergine (eggplant), discard the seeds and chop the flesh into small dice.

In a bowl, mix the aubergine (eggplant), onion and peppers with the olive oil, parsley, sherry vinegar and salt. Finely chop the anchovies and stir in at the last moment. Transfer to a serving dish.

Toss the almonds in the smoked paprika and sprinkle over the roasted vegetables. Garnish with the reserved onion.

Note: This is a great dish – it can also be cooked in the foil over hot coals on a barbecue for a wonderful smoky flavour and aroma. Just use a double layer of foil and it will take about 1 hour.

NUTRITION FACTS

Anchovies contain one of the most dense amounts of the beneficial Omega-3 essential fats, used by the body for gut healing and repair, as well as an anti-inflammatory nutrient for heart health.

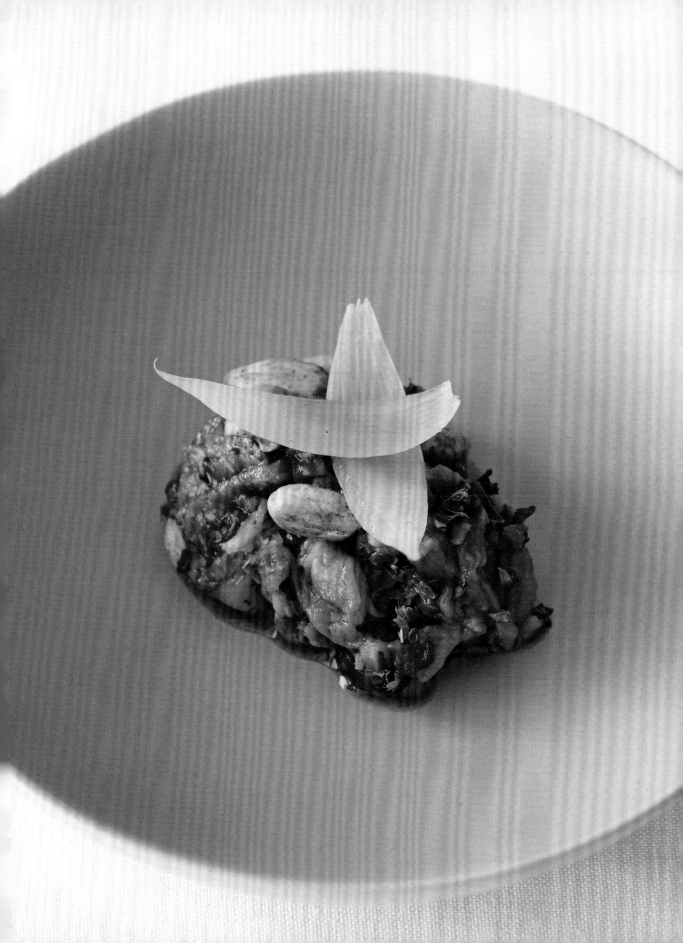

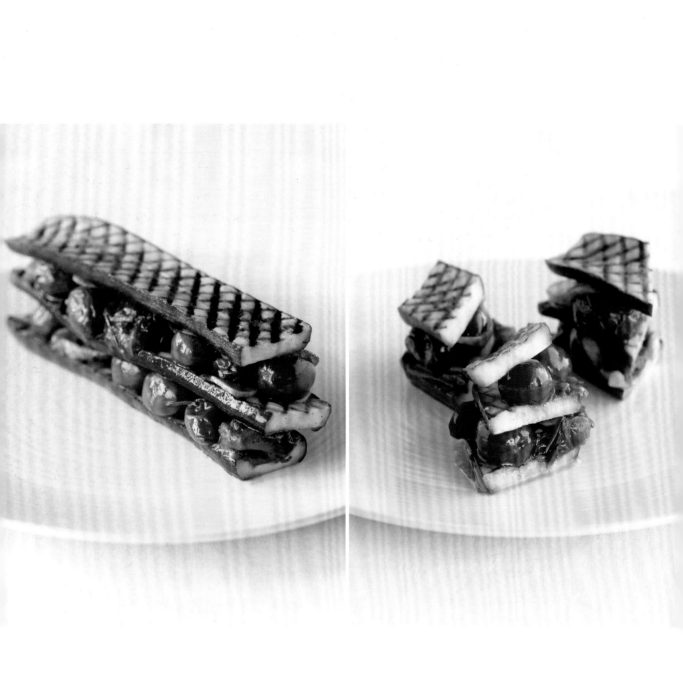

(P) Grilled courgettes with slow-roasted cherry tomatoes & shallots

Shallots are more intensely flavoured than onions and tend to be sweeter when cooked. These classic Mediterranean vegetables are simple to prepare. Griddling the courgettes (zucchini) ensures that they maintain their crunch and provide a contrast to the juicy tomatoes from the oven.

Serves 4

500g (1lb 2oz) mixed cherry tomatoes
100g (3½oz) shallots, thinly sliced
2 garlic cloves, peeled
10g (½oz) rosemary sprigs
pinch of salt
ground black pepper
20g (¾oz) clarified butter
2 large courgettes (zucchini), sliced lengthways 1cm (½in) thick
juice of ½ lemon

Preheat the oven to 150°C, 300°F, Gas mark 2.

Place the tomatoes, shallots, garlic, rosemary, salt, black pepper and half the clarified butter in an ovenproof dish. Mix together, and then slow-roast in the preheated oven for 40–50 minutes until the tomatoes are cooked and their skins have split.

Meanwhile, heat a ridged griddle pan over a high heat. Arrange the courgettes (zucchini) on a large tray, drizzle with the remaining butter, and season with salt and pepper and a squeeze of lemon juice. Grill them in batches in the hot pan for 1 minute on each side until cooked.

Layer the grilled courgettes (zucchini) with the warm roasted tomatoes to serve.

CHEF'S TIP
Slow-roasting helps to preserve the moisture of all vegetables, bringing out their natural sweetness as well as guarding their nutrients.

Post-Plan vegetable side dishes

The post-Plan addition of some of the denser root vegetables, including parsnips and sweet potato, adds a natural sweetness to the following recipes as well as expanding the variety and range of vegetable side dishes that you can now eat. The inclusion of further pulses, such as chickpeas, broadens the possibilities of different vegetable combinations.

P+ Parsnips roasted with mustard, honey & thyme

Owing to their complex structure and the difficulty of breaking them down in a resting gut, these humble root vegetables should be saved for the post-Plan stage. This is a classic recipe brought alive by the addition of thyme, which imparts its distinctive aroma on roasting.

Serves 4

2 tbsp local runny honey
1 tsp English mustard
1 tsp clarified butter
pinch of salt
ground black pepper
500g (1lb 2oz) parsnips, peeled, quartered and tough core removed
1 bunch of fresh thyme

Preheat the oven to 180°C, 350°F, Gas mark 4. Line a baking sheet with some silicone paper.

In a large bowl, mix together the honey, mustard, butter, salt and pepper. Add the cut parsnips and turn them in the mixture. Sprinkle the whole sprigs of thyme onto the baking sheet and then lay the parsnips on top.

Roast in the preheated oven for about 20–25 minutes, turning the parsnips after 15 minutes.

Serve the parsnips in a warmed vegetable dish on top of the thyme.

NUTRITION FACTS

This sweeter-than-most root vegetable is rich in B vitamins for energy and antioxidants that help the body neutralize toxins. Parsnips are high in soluble and insoluble fibre, and make a great addition to any dish when balancing bitter and sweet flavours.

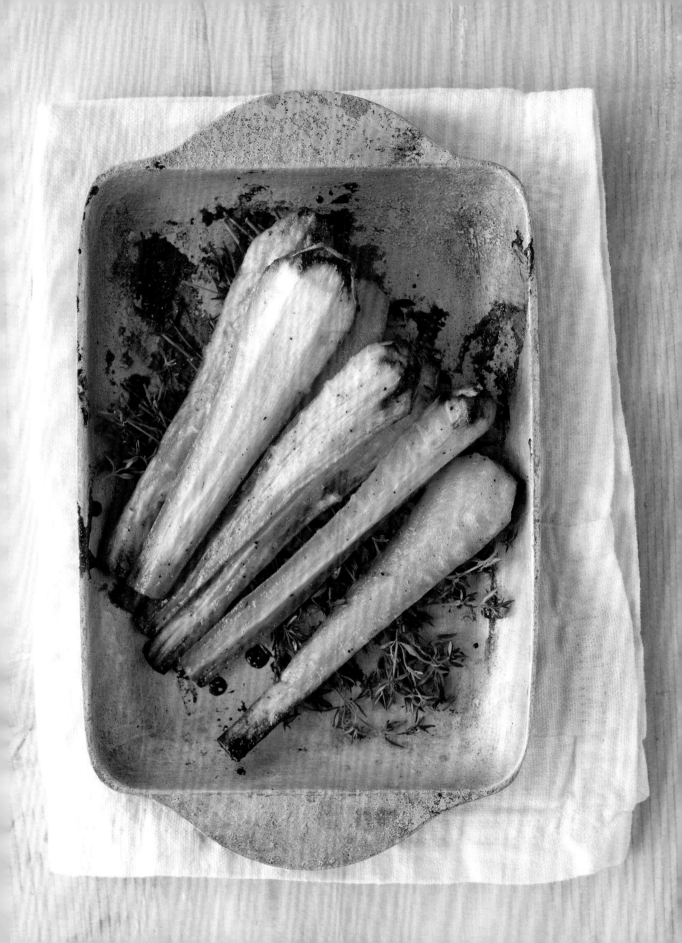

P+ Sweet potato & chickpea cakes with lime & cucumber raita

Sweet potatoes are another root vegetable saved for the post-Plan phase. They add natural sweetness to any dish. These chickpea cakes are easy to make and can be frozen. Make them a staple food in your weekly meal plans, as they are just as delicious when eaten cold.

Serves 4

20g (¾oz) butter

140g (4½oz) onion, finely chopped

1 garlic clove, crushed

20g (¾oz) fresh root ginger, peeled and finely chopped

1 small fresh red chilli, deseeded and finely chopped

½ tsp hot curry powder

80g (3oz/½ cup) chickpeas, soaked overnight in acidulated water, cooked and drained

250g (8oz) sweet potato, peeled and grated

10g (½oz) coriander (cilantro), roughly chopped

juice of ½ lemon

fresh lemon wedges, to serve

For the lime & cucumber raita:

50g (2oz) cucumber, grated

150g (5oz/1¼ cups) 24-hour fermented yoghurt (see page 52)

grated zest of ½ lime

a few spinach leaves, chopped

2 tsp local runny honey

pinch of Lime zest, kaffir lime and lemongrass salt (see page 36)

few mint sprigs, chopped

Preheat the oven to 180°C, 350°F, Gas mark 4.

In a thick-bottomed pan, melt the butter and sauté the onion, garlic, ginger and chilli until golden brown. Add the curry powder and 4 teaspoons of cold water (to stop the curry powder burning). Cook for 1 minute, then add the cooked chickpeas, crushing them slightly with the back of a spoon. Add the sweet potato and lemon juice. Continue cooking for 2–3 minutes until the sweet potato releases some starch and the mixture starts to stick together.

Remove the pan from the heat and stir in the coriander (cilantro). Take portions of the mixture and, using your hands, form them into 8 little cakes. Place them on a parchment-lined baking sheet.

Cook in the preheated oven for 12 minutes, turning the cakes over after 6 minutes, until golden brown on both sides.

While the cakes are cooking, make the raita. Mix all the ingredients together in a small bowl.

Serve the warm potato and chickpea cakes with a side dish of raita and some fresh lime wedges.

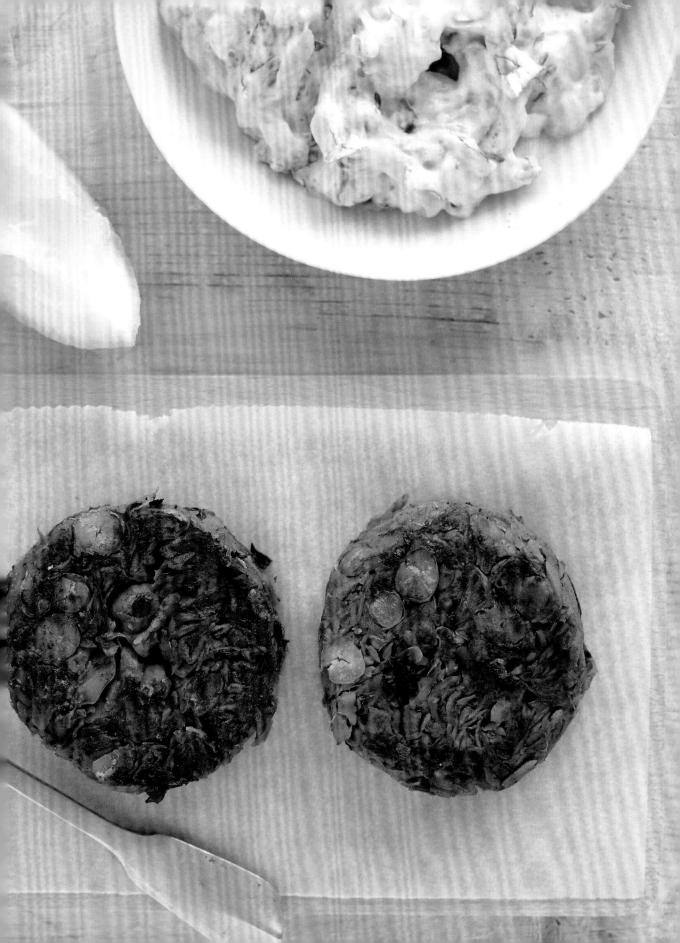

P+ Pea, feta & sesame lollipops with mint yoghurt sauce

There's a lot going on in these delicious treats, with protein from the different cheeses, sesame seeds, gram flour (chick pea flour), peas and the yoghurt dip, all bursting with a fresh tangy flavour. Make these lollipops in large batches, as they will disappear faster than you expect.

Serves 4

250g (8oz/2 cups) cooked garden peas

125g (4oz) feta cheese

10g (½oz) mint leaves, chopped

1 fresh green chilli, deseeded and finely chopped

30g (1¼oz/¼ cup) grated Parmesan

2 organic free-range egg yolks

½ tsp chilli powder

30g (1¼oz/¼ cup) gram (chick pea) flour

sesame seeds, for sprinkling

60g (2½oz) coconut oil

For the radish salad:

1 tsp hazelnut oil

1 tsp sherry vinegar

½ tsp local runny honey

60g (2½oz) radishes, thinly sliced

10 mint leaves, finely shredded

For the mint yoghurt sauce:

100ml (3½fl oz) 24-hour fermented yoghurt (see page 52), strained in a coffee filter to a Greek-style consistency

1 fresh red chilli, deseeded and finely chopped

pinch of saffron

pinch of salt

1 tbsp chopped mint

½ tsp local runny honey

Use a stick blender to blend the peas, feta cheese, mint, fresh chilli, Parmesan, egg yolks and chilli powder. The mixture does not need to be really smooth – a few lumps are fine. Pour into a large mixing bowl and stir in the gram flour to tighten up the mixture.

With your hands, roll pieces of the mixture into 8 equal-sized balls. Flatten them a little and skewer with a lollipop stick. Sprinkle with sesame seeds and arrange them on a plate lined with greaseproof paper. Keep in the fridge until ready to cook.

Make the radish salad: whisk together the oil, vinegar and honey to make a dressing for the radishes. Toss lightly with the radishes and arrange on a plate. Sprinkle with the shredded mint.

Make the mint yoghurt sauce: gently stir all the ingredients together in a small bowl. Do not whisk them as the yoghurt will break up and become too runny.

To cook the lollipops, heat the coconut oil in a small pan and then shallow-fry them, turning occasionally, until they are golden brown and hot in the centre.

Serve the lollipops on the radish salad with the mint yoghurt sauce in a side dish for dipping.

CHEF'S TIP

Children will love these, too, and it's a great way to get them eating the essential fats and flavours you wouldn't normally expect them to devour.

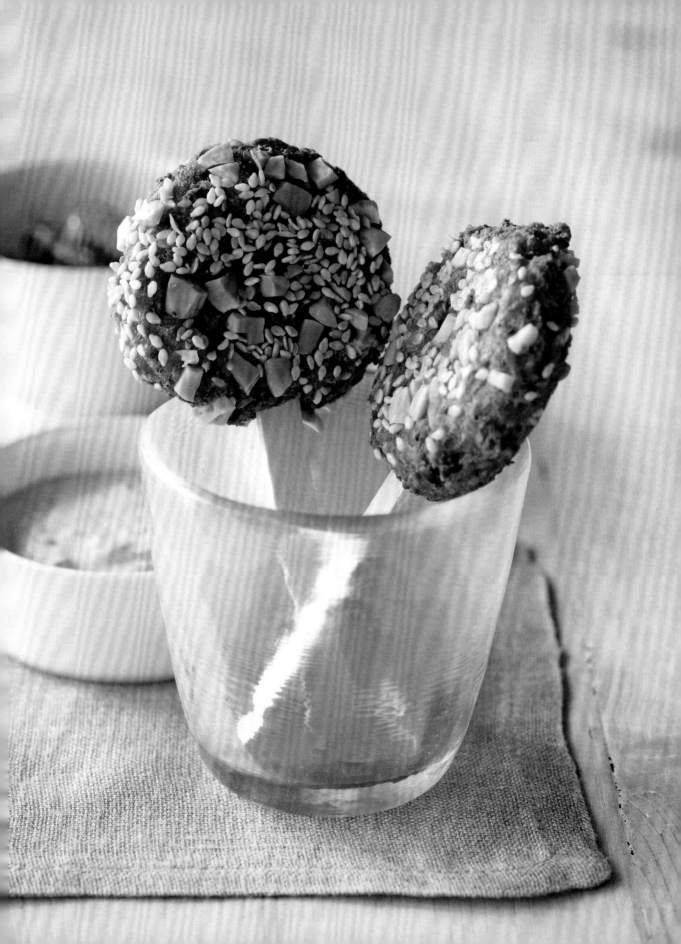

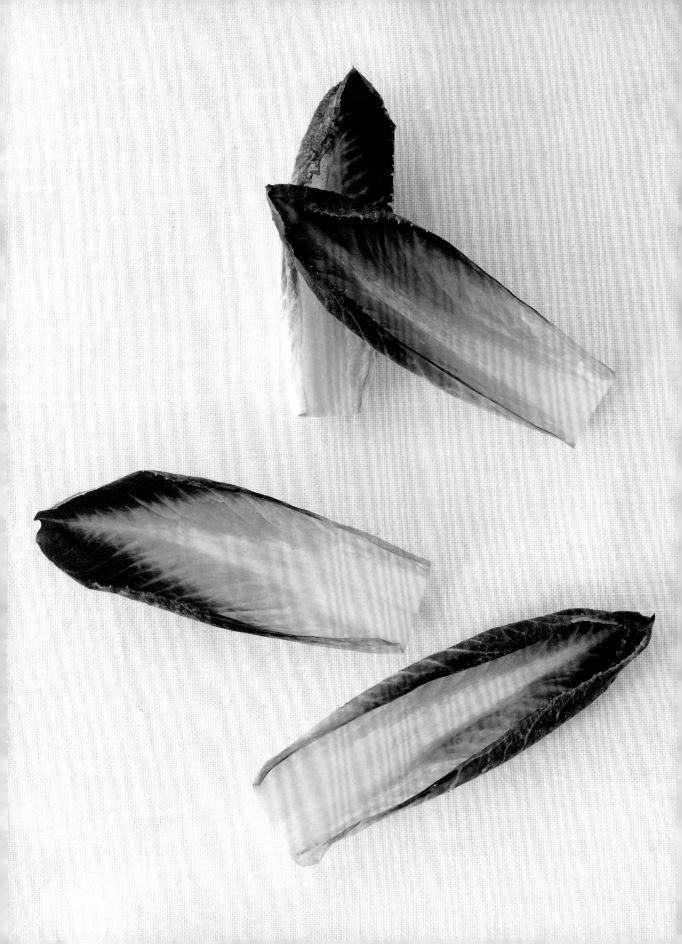

Salads

Blanched salads

The following salads have been compiled from various groups of vegetables, half of which have been blanched to break down their cellulose. This is to ensure that they are more easily digested in the resting gut. It's a key element of the principles of the Good Gut, Great Health Plan, where the vegetables and salad ingredients are chosen for their range of nutrients rather than their high degree of dietary fibre. Many of the ingredients can be prepared and bagged in advance to put in the fridge for easy assembly when required. The essence is to combine vegetables and leaves for their colour and texture, so freshness of ingredients is key. The ability to mix and match the salads with the dressings is the joy of this Plan.

The vegetables are sliced, shredded or diced, then flash-blanched for just 5 seconds before being refreshed in iced water to keep them really crisp with a crunchy texture. The next step is to add nuts, seeds, coconut, herbs and other ingredients as well as salad leaves and toss everything lightly together with the dressing of your choice. For each salad, we suggest a dressing that perfectly matches the combination of blanched vegetables/seeds/nuts/herbs, but the beauty of preparing salads like these is that you can mix and match any of the combinations according to your personal taste. Give them a try and start creating your own combinations. Remember that all the flavour is in the dressing. Always dress the salad just before you are ready to eat it as the vegetables will become soggy if dressed too early.

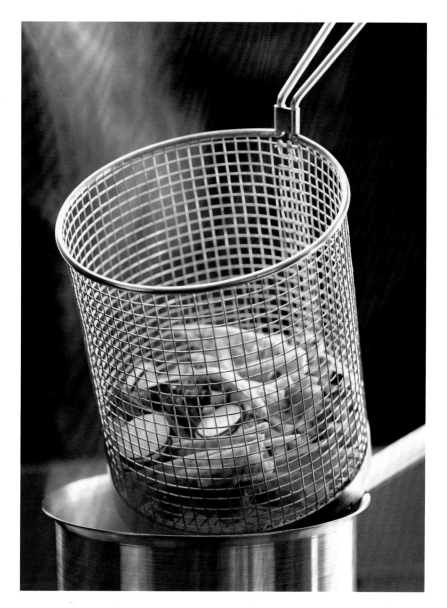

Above: To blanch salad vegeteables, add them to boiling water for 5 seconds.
Opposite: Remove and drain the vegetables before immersing them in iced water.

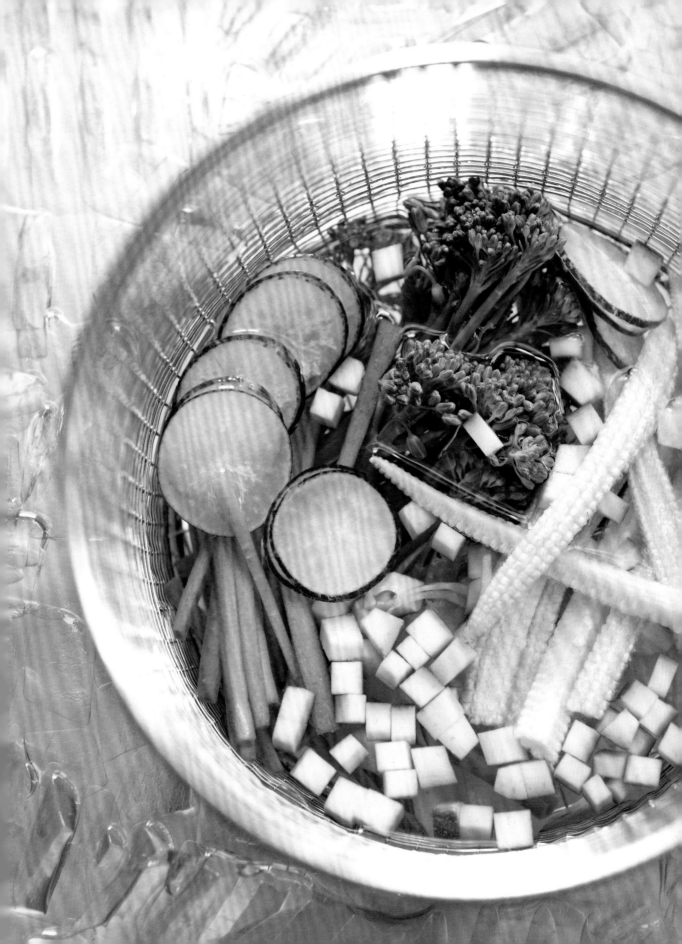

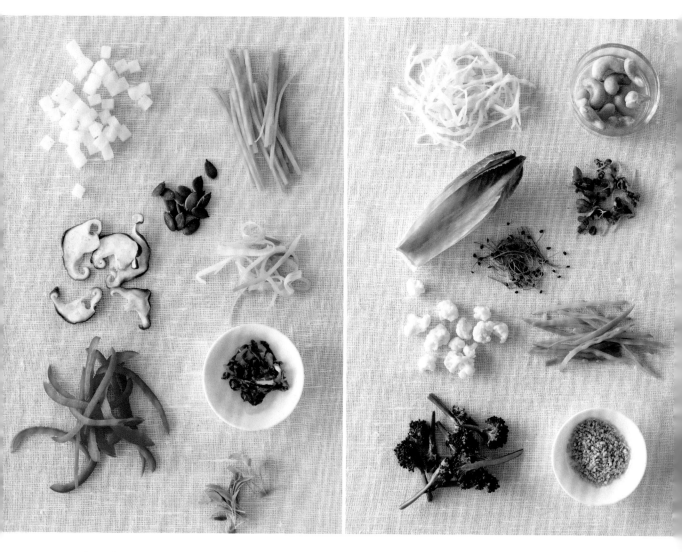

Ingredients for Blanched salad (1)

Ingredients for Blanched salad (2)

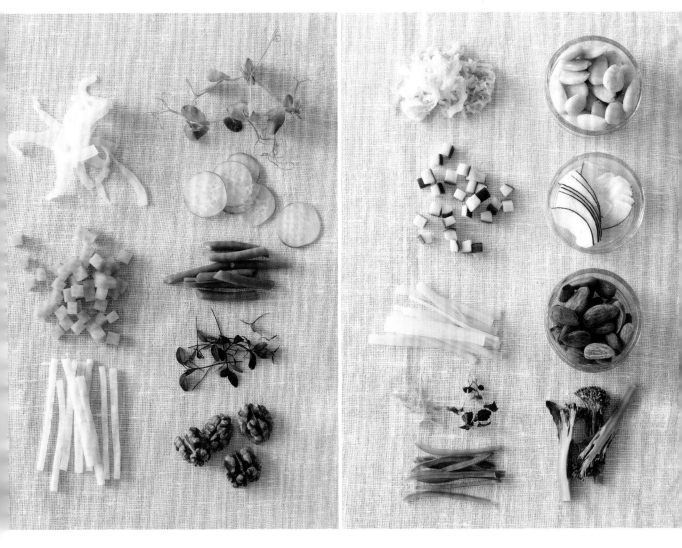

Ingredients for Blanched salad (3)   Ingredients for Blanched salad (4)

P Blanched salad (1)

The secret is to have all the ingredients ready prepared to plunge into boiling water at the same time to ensure that nothing wilts and the colours are retained. Choose only the freshest sprouted pumpkin seeds or use seeds that have been soaked. The coriander (cilantro) and mint are key.

Serves 4

70g (2¾oz) shiitake mushrooms, sliced

80g (3oz) red (bell) pepper, cored, deseeded and cut into fine strips

80g (3oz) carrot, cut into fine strips

80g (3oz) pak choi, shredded

2 spring onions (scallions), shredded

100g (3½oz) mouli, cut into fine strips

For sprinkling:

10g (½oz) pumpkin seeds, soaked overnight in cold water

baby coriander (cilantro), for sprinkling

few mint sprigs, shredded

For the suggested dressing:

90ml (3½fl oz/¹/₃ cup) Mango, lemongrass, ginger, mint & coriander dressing (see page 211)

Prepare all the vegetables as directed. Blanch them in a pan of boiling water for just 5 seconds. Drain in a colander and refresh immediately by plunging them into a bowl of iced water. Remove and then dry thoroughly on kitchen paper.

Mix the vegetables in a large bowl with the dressing.

Serve on a plate sprinkled with the soaked pumpkin seeds, baby coriander (cilantro) and mint.

NUTRITION FACTS

The advantage of blanching vegetables is that it breaks down their cellulose content without leaching any of their essential nutrients.

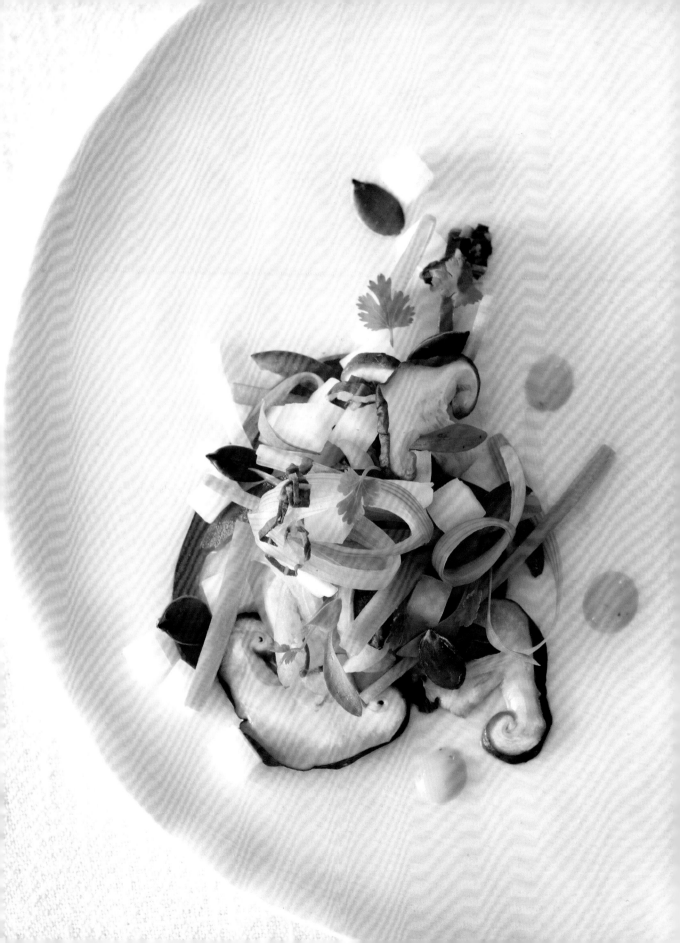

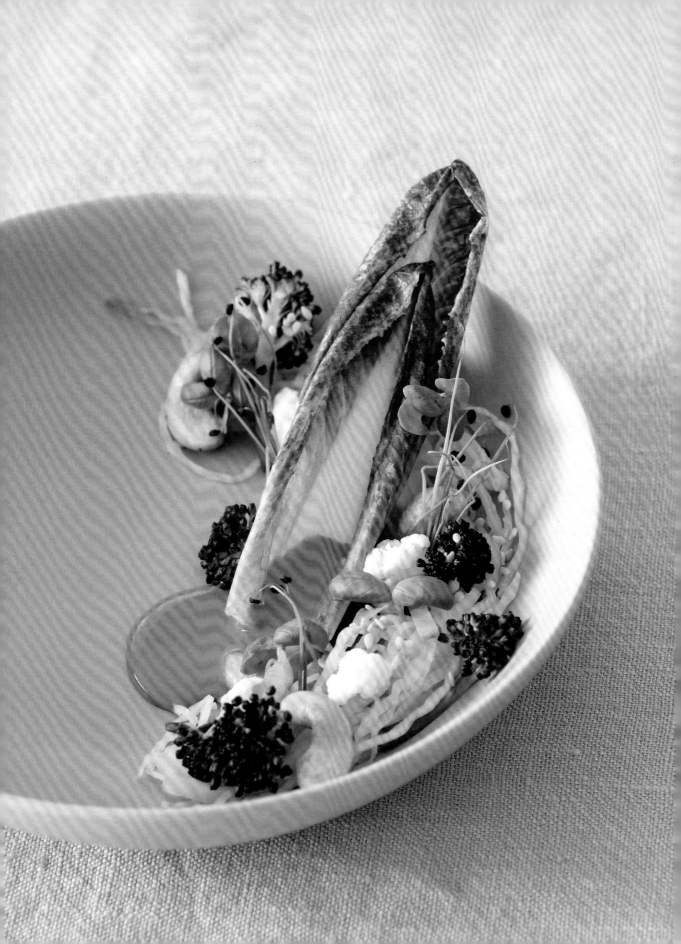

(P) Blanched salad (2)

Chicory (Belgian endive) can have a bitter taste but here it is balanced beautifully with the mangetout, cabbage and cauliflower florets to provide a substantial salad. The addition of soaked cashews and sesame seeds provides the protein content in this brassica vegetable salad.

Serves 4

100g (3½oz) red chicory (Belgian endive)

100g (3½oz) very small cauliflower florets

100g (3½oz) mangetout, cut into fine strips

100g (3½oz) white cabbage, finely shredded

100g (3½oz) purple sprouting broccoli, cut into thirds lengthways

5g (¼oz) toasted sesame seeds

60g (2½oz/¾ cup) cashew nuts, soaked in cold water overnight

For sprinkling:

10g (½oz) baby basil

5g (¼oz) rock chives

For the suggested dressing:

90ml (3½fl oz/⅓ cup) Raspberry, wasabi, tahini & maple dressing (see page 212)

Prepare all the vegetables as directed. Blanch them in a pan of boiling water for just 5 seconds. Drain in a colander and refresh immediately by plunging them into a bowl of iced water. Remove and then dry thoroughly on kitchen paper.

In a large bowl, gently toss the blanched vegetables, sesame seeds and cashew nuts in the dressing.

Serve on a plate, sprinkled with baby basil and rock chives.

NUTRITION FACTS

Cashew nuts provide the protein content in this salad, being creamy but crunchy when soaked, and packed with magnesium, for heart health, manganese for bones and ligaments, and zinc for immunity. A nutrient-dense powerhouse of a food.

P Blanched salad (3)

Fennel, radishes and celeriac all have a subtle tinge of licorice flavour, which is offset by the sweetness of the green beans and the creamy crunch of the walnuts. Top this off with the diced butternut squash and you have a veritable rainbow of vegetables on your plate.

Serves 4

100g (3½oz) fennel bulb, finely sliced

100g (3½oz) butternut squash, peeled and cut into 5mm (⅛in) dice

100g (3½oz) radishes, sliced

100g (3½oz) celeriac, peeled and cut into fine strips

100g (3½oz) fine green beans, trimmed and cut in half

80g (3oz/1 cup) walnuts, soaked in cold water overnight

For sprinkling:

80g (3oz) pea shoots

40g (1½oz) red amaranth

For the suggested dressing:

90ml (3½fl oz/⅓ cup) Walnut, tarragon, shallot & honey dressing (see page 212)

Prepare all the vegetables as directed. Blanch them in a pan of boiling water for just 5 seconds. Drain in a colander and refresh immediately by plunging them into a bowl of iced water. Remove the vegetables and then dry thoroughly on kitchen paper.

In a large bowl, gently toss the vegetables and walnuts together with the dressing.

Serve on a plate with pea shoots and red amaranth sprinkled on top.

NUTRITION FACTS

Walnuts provide one of the richest available sources of Omega-3, to assist healing and repair of the gut, brain and heart health, thick luscious hair and supple skin.

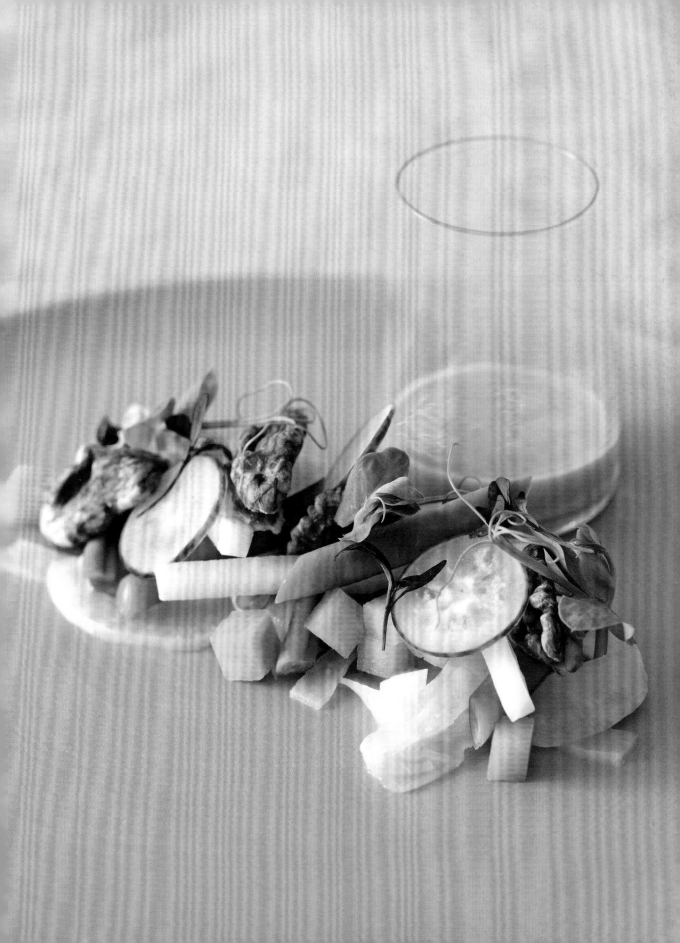

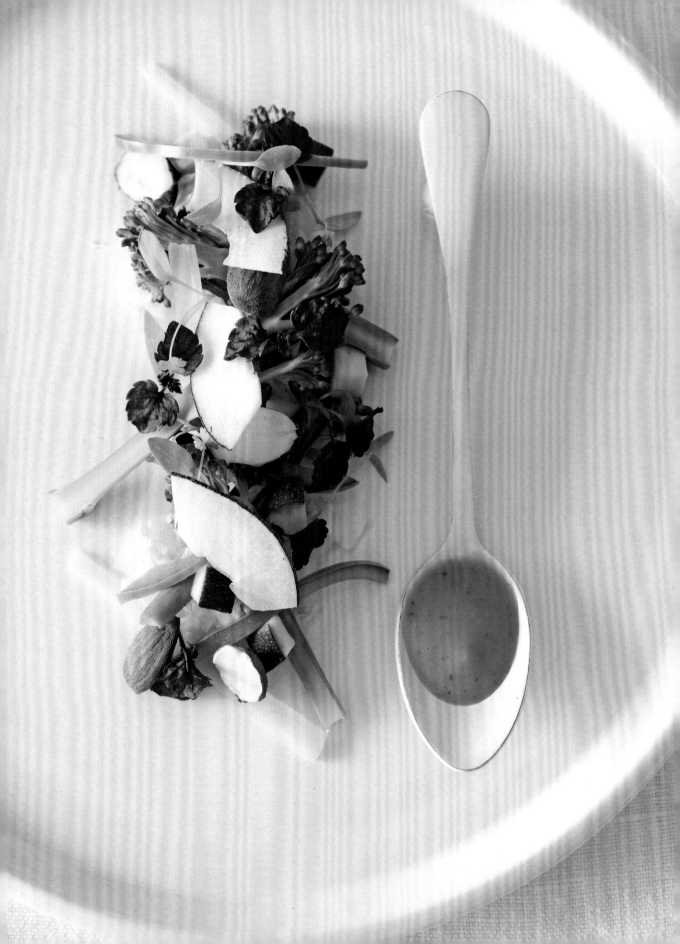

(P) Blanched salad (4)

Tenderstem broccoli has made a huge impact on the vegetables we eat on a regular basis, and rightly so, as it is full of flavour and the stems are more digestible than the larger heads of calabrese. Celery has a naturally salty flavour but tastes really fresh in this blanched form.

Serves 4

100g (3½oz) Chinese leaf (napa), finely shredded

100g (3½oz) courgette (zucchini), cut into 3mm (⅛in) dice

80g (3oz) celery, peeled and finely sliced

125g (4oz) tenderstem broccoli, each cut in half lengthways and then into 3 long pieces

100g (3½oz) green (bell) pepper, deseeded and cut into fine strips

For sprinkling:

60g (2oz/scant ½ cup) whole almonds, soaked overnight in cold water

10g (½oz) coconut flakes, soaked overnight

20g (¾oz) Shiso cress

10g (½oz) baby celery leaf

For the suggested dressing:

90ml (3½fl oz/⅓ cup) Roasted pineapple, kumquat & five-spice dressing (see page 213)

Prepare all the vegetables as directed. Blanch them in a pan of boiling water for just 5 seconds. Drain in a colander and then refresh immediately by plunging them into a bowl of iced water. Remove and the vegetables and then dry thoroughly on kitchen paper.

Transfer the prepared vegetables to a large mixing bowl and toss them gently in the dressing.

Serve on a plate sprinkled with almonds, flaked coconut, Shiso cress and celery leaves.

NUTRITION FACTS

Tenderstem broccoli is packed with beta-carotene and vitamin C, two of the essential antioxidants that the body requires daily, as well as folic acid, which is vital for the nervous and neurological systems.

Salad dressings

A salad is not complete without its dressing and the beauty of the six that have been created here is that any one of them may be eaten with any of the four salads on the Plan and also the post-Plan salads. Each may be stored in jars or bottles in the fridge for up to 3–4 days as they have no preservatives and really are so much more delicious than commercial varieties. Using a hand or jug blender increases the amount of air, thereby creating a light yet creamy dressing.

Raspberry, wasabi, tahini
& maple dressing

Mango, lemongrass, ginger, mint
& coriander dressing

Roasted pineapple, kumquat
& five-spice dressing

P Mango, lemongrass, ginger, mint & coriander dressing

Serves 10

1 large ripe mango, peeled, stoned and roughly chopped

2 lemongrass stalks, peeled and finely chopped

2cm (1in) piece of fresh root ginger, peeled and chopped

1 tbsp cider vinegar

100ml (3½fl oz/generous ⅓ cup) sunflower oil (cold pressed)

juice of 1 lime

15g (½oz) fresh mint leaves

15g (½oz) coriander (cilantro)

1 fresh green chilli, deseeded and finely chopped

To make the dressing, you'll need either a stick blender or a jug blender.

Simply blend all the ingredients together until smooth and emulsified.

If possible, leave the dressing for at least 30 minutes to allow the flavours to combine and maximize the different layers of flavour from the herbs and lemongrass.

Pass the dressing through a fine sieve and store in a sterilized screwtop jar in the fridge for up to 5 days.

Walnut, tarragon, shallot & honey dressing

Chilli, lime, papaya & mint dressing

Roasted red pepper, tomato, garlic & paprika dressing

P Chilli, lime, papaya & mint dressing

Serves 10

1 fresh small red chilli, deseeded and finely sliced

1 tsp grated lime zest

5 tsp lime juice

few coriander (cilantro) sprigs, chopped

300g (10oz) papaya, peeled, deseeded and chopped

10g (½oz) mint leaves, chopped

80ml (3fl oz/scant ⅓ cup) olive oil

Put all the ingredients in a food processor and blend until smooth.

Pass the dressing through a fine sieve, pressing it down well with the back of a spoon.

Store the dressing in a sterilized screwtop jar in the fridge for up to 5 days.

P Raspberry, wasabi, tahini & maple dressing

Serves 8

300g (10oz/2½ cups) fresh or frozen raspberries

100ml (3½fl oz/generous ⅓ cup) cider vinegar

25g (1oz) tahini

7 tsp pure maple syrup

4 tsp toasted sesame oil

70ml (2½fl oz/generous ¼ cup) cold-pressed olive oil

10g (½oz) wasabi paste

50ml (2fl oz/scant ¼ cup) water

To make the dressing, you will need a stick blender or a jug blender.

Blend all the ingredients together until smooth and then pass the dressing through a fine sieve into a sterilized jar with a screwtop lid. The dressing can be kept in the fridge for up to 5 days.

Note: This dressing is very stable but a slight separation may occur; if so, simply shake or whisk to emulsify again.

P Walnut, tarragon, shallot & honey dressing

Serves 10

50g (2oz/½ cup) walnut pieces, soaked for at least 12 hours

100ml (3½fl oz/generous ⅓ cup) walnut oil

50ml (2fl oz/scant ¼ cup) extra virgin olive oil

3 sprigs of tarragon, stalks removed

5g (¼oz) chervil, roughly chopped

10g (½ oz) basil leaves

2 tbsp cider vinegar

2 tbsp Dijon mustard

1 shallot, roughly chopped

juice of ½ lemon

30g (1oz) local runny honey

Thoroughly rinse the soaked walnuts under running cold water and then drain well.

Using a stick or a jug blender, blitz the remaining ingredients until emulsified. Pass through a fine sieve into a sterilized jar with a screwtop lid and keep in the fridge for up to 5 days.

Note: If the dressing separates, shake the jar, or whisk back into an emulsion.

P Roasted red pepper, tomato, garlic & paprika dressing

Serves 10

200g (7oz) ripe red tomatoes

1 large red (bell) pepper

1 tsp fennel seeds

½ tsp cumin seeds

1 tsp coriander seeds

100ml (3½fl oz/generous ⅓ cup) chia oil

2 garlic cloves, thinly sliced

5 tsp cider vinegar

20g (¾oz) local runny honey

pinch of sea salt

½ tsp smoked sweet paprika

pinch of cayenne pepper

Preheat the oven to 220°C, 425°F, Gas mark 7.

Cut the tomatoes in half and place them on a baking tray with the whole red (bell) pepper. Roast in the preheated oven for 25 minutes or until the skin blisters on the pepper and the tomatoes start to burn slightly on top.

Remove from the oven and leave to cool. Skin the pepper, remove the seeds and roughly chop the flesh. Squeeze some of the seeds out of the tomatoes and discard them (this will make the dressing sweeter).

In a small dry pan, toast the fennel, cumin and coriander seeds over a low heat until they start to release their natural aromas. Add 1 tsp of the chia oil and the garlic and gently toast until the garlic turns golden brown. Do not let it burn or it will become very bitter.

Using either a stick blender or a jug blender, blitz all the ingredients to a smooth emulsion. Pass through a fine sieve into a sterilized jar with a screwtop lid and keep refrigerated for up to 5 days.

P Roasted pineapple, kumquat & five-spice dressing

Serves 10

300g (10oz) ripe pineapple, peeled, cored and cut into 1cm (½in) chunks

50g (2oz) kumquats, cut in half

25g (1oz) local runny honey

pinch of five-spice powder

finely grated zest and juice of ½ lime

5 tsp cider vinegar

100ml (3½fl oz/generous ⅓ cup) avocado oil

50ml (2fl oz/scant ¼ cup) water

Preheat the oven to 200°C, 400°F, Gas mark 6.

Line a small roasting tray with parchment paper. Place the pineapple and kumquats on the tray and drizzle with the honey.

Roast in the preheated oven for 20–25 minutes until the fruit has caramelized. Remove from the oven and set aside to cool.

Using either a stick blender or a jug blender, blend the roasted fruit with all the remaining ingredients until smooth and emulsified.

Pass through a fine sieve into a sterilized jar with a screwtop lid and keep in the fridge for up to 5 days.

Note: If the dressing separates, just shake the jar vigorously until it emulsifies.

Post-Plan salads

These post-Plan salads are more substantial as they allow additional ingredients, including sweet potato, some cheeses and grains, such as wild rice, that were not included in the Plan. These salads are a meal in themselves and can be eaten for lunch or supper, depending on how busy you are. Unlike the salads on the Plan, the vegetables need not be blanched.

P+ Sweet potato salad with mango & puffed wild rice

Wild rice is actually seaweed and not a grain and it's absolutely delicious when it is cooked in coconut oil. The inclusion of shaved fennel adds an aniseed edge to the relative sweetness of the antioxidant-rich sweet potato, mango and apricots.

Serves 4

300g (10oz) sweet potato, peeled and cut into 1cm (½in) cubes

4 unsulphured dried apricots, cut into fine strips

6 spring onions (scallions), chopped

10g (½oz) fresh coriander (cilantro), chopped

20g (¾oz) coconut oil

40g (1½oz) wild rice, cooked in boiling water for 25 minutes, then drained and dried on kitchen paper

1 small fennel bulb, shaved on a mandolin, then covered with cold water and left in the fridge for 1 hour

For the dressing:

2 tbsp olive oil

1 fresh red chilli, deseeded and roughly chopped

2.5cm (1in) piece of fresh root ginger, peeled and roughly chopped

1 large mango, peeled, stoned and cut into 5mm (¼in) dice

1 tsp roasted curry powder

1 tbsp chopped fresh coriander (cilantro)

1 tbsp local runny honey

75ml (3fl oz) 24-hour fermented yoghurt (see page 52)

Cook the sweet potato in a pan of boiling water for 15 minutes until soft. Refresh under cold running water. Drain in a colander.

Make the dressing: blitz the olive oil, chilli, ginger, half the diced mango, curry powder, coriander (cilantro) and honey in a jug blender until you have a smooth paste. Pass it through a fine strainer into a mixing bowl. Gently stir in the yoghurt – do not whisk as it will separate and the dressing will be too thick.

Put the sweet potato, remaining mango, apricots, spring onions (scallions) and coriander (cilantro) in a large bowl. Add the dressing and mix thoroughly. Spoon onto serving plates.

To puff the wild rice, heat the coconut oil in a small pan set over a medium heat. When hot, add the cooked wild rice and fry for 30 seconds until it puffs up. Remove immediately with a slotted spoon and drain on kitchen paper.

Drain the crunchy shaved fennel in a colander and scatter over the sweet potato salad. Sprinkle with the puffed wild rice.

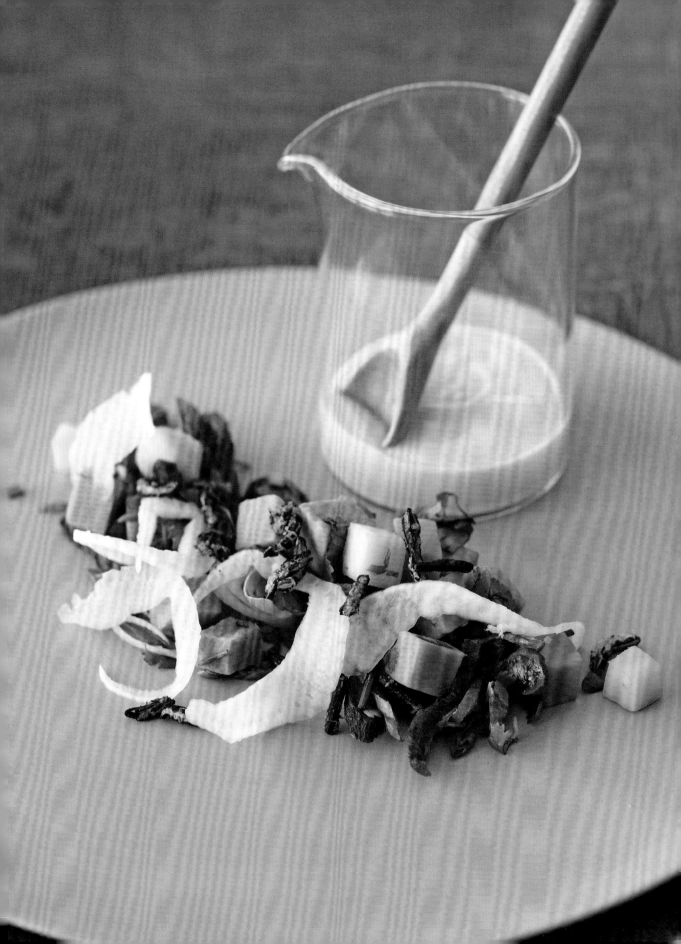

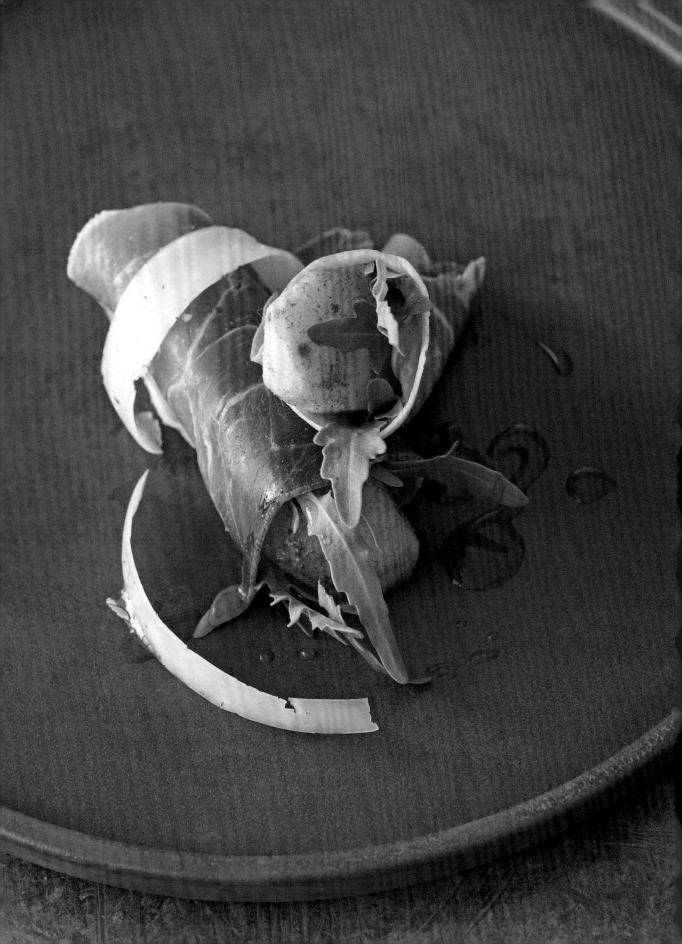

P+ Spiced pear with serrano ham & manchego

In this delicious twist on a classic Italian dish, the pears have a natural sweetness, which, when baked with hot paprika and mixed spice, creates the perfect accompaniment to the saltiness of the Serrano ham and the Manchego cheese, which is made from sheep's milk.

Serves 4

2 tsp local runny honey

½ tsp hot paprika (picante)

½ tsp mixed spice

3 tsp aged sherry vinegar

juice of ½ lemon

3 ripe Conference pears

12 thin slices Serrano ham

100g (3½oz) baby rocket (arugula) leaves plus extra for garnish

50g (2oz) Manchego cheese, sliced thinly with a potato peeler

Preheat the oven to 180°C, 350°F, Gas mark 4.

In a large mixing bowl, mix the honey, paprika, mixed spice, sherry vinegar and lemon juice.

Peel the pears and cut into quarters, removing the cores and stalks. Add them to the spicy paprika marinade and turn them gently to coat them all over with then mixture.

Line a baking sheet with parchment paper and arrange the pears on top. Roast in the preheated oven for 12–15 minutes. Remove and allow to cool, saving the cooking juices.

Place a slice of Serrano ham on a chopping board. Gather a few baby rocket (arugula)leaves into a small bunch and place on top of the ham. Top with a cooked pear and then roll up. Repeat with the remaining ham, rocket and pears.

Arrange the ham rolls on 4 serving plates and drizzle with the reserved cooking juices. Garnish with baby rocket (arugula) and shaved Manchego cheese.

NUTRITION FACTS

Pears are a rich source of peptin, which helps to remove toxins from the gut.

P+ Sprouting seeds & lentils with roasted peaches & kale

The protein potential in sprouted seeds is unrivalled and balances this salad by providing a crunchy vegetarian alternative. Ruby chard and kale have a very high calcium, iron and magnesium content to cleanse the digestion and provide energy for the body.

Serves 4

4 ripe peaches or nectarines, stoned and each cut into 6 wedges

250g (8oz) sprouting seeds and sprouting lentils

30g (1¼oz) red lentils, soaked in boiling water for 20 minutes, then drained

50g (2oz) curly kale, blanched in boiling water for 40 seconds, then refreshed in iced water

50g (2oz) baby red chard, washed

For the dressing:

2 tbsp olive oil

4 tsp cider vinegar

juice of ½ lemon

4 tsp maple syrup

1 fresh red chilli, deseeded and roughly chopped

10g (½oz) mint leaves

Preheat the oven to 200°C, 400°F, Gas mark 6.

Line a baking sheet with parchment paper and place the peaches or nectarines on top. Bake in the preheated oven for 15 minutes until soft. Remove and set aside to cool on the tray.

Make the dressing: blitz one-third of the roasted peaches in a jug blender with the remaining dressing ingredients until smooth. Pass the dressing through a fine sieve into a clean bowl.

On a large serving platter, scatter the sprouting lentils and seeds and red lentils. Neatly lay the roasted peaches on top, and sprinkle with the blanched curly kale and baby chard leaves. Drizzle the dressing over the salad just before serving.

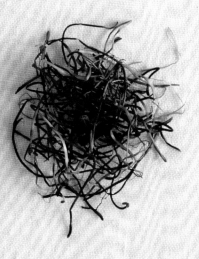

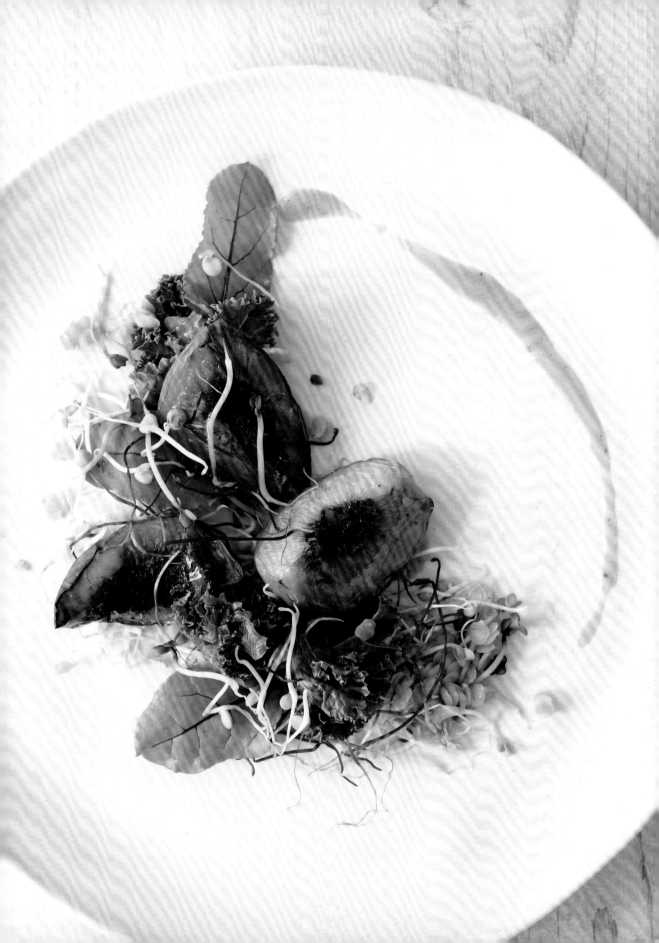

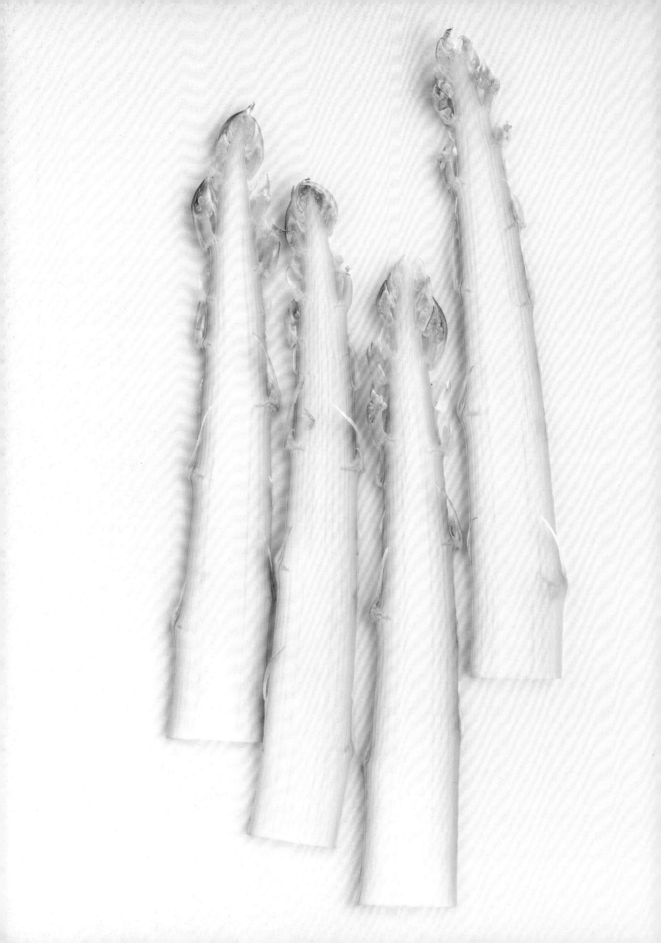

Special occasions

(P) Lamb with grilled asparagus and salsa verde

This unusual marinade uses anchovy fillets to flavour red meat and, surprisingly, it works a treat. The trick is to undercook the lamb and allow it to rest – this ensures that the meat remains juicy, tender, succulent and pink. The richness of the colour is an indicator of the nutrient density of red meat.

Serves 8–10

4 x 125g (4oz) pieces lamb loin, fully trimmed and all sinews removed

20g (¾oz/1½ tbsp) clarified butter

2 bundles of asparagus, trimmed and cut in half

1 tsp chia oil

For the marinade:

2 garlic cloves, crushed

3 rosemary sprigs, chopped

grated zest of ½ lemon

1 tsp local runny honey

For the salsa verde:

25g (1oz) mint leaves

25g (1oz) basil leaves

25g (1oz) flat-leaf parsley

1 garlic clove, crushed

3 spring onions (scallions)

1 tbsp capers

8 anchovy fillets

1 tsp Dijon mustard

2 tbsp extra virgin olive oil

sea salt and ground black pepper

Mix together all the marinade ingredients in a bowl. Add the lamb, then cover and leave to marinate for 2 hours in the fridge.

Make the salsa verde, put all the ingredients in a blender and blitz until smooth. Keep in a screwtop jar in the fridge for up to 1 week.

Preheat the oven to 200°C, 400°F, Gas mark 6.

Heat the clarified butter in a small frying pan over a high heat. Remove some of the marinade from the lamb and then add the lamb to the hot pan and sear it on all sides. Season with some sea salt and black pepper, and then roast in the preheated oven for 5 minutes until pink. Remove and allow to rest.

Heat a griddle pan over a high heat. In a bowl, drizzle the asparagus with the chia oil. Season with salt and pepper and then arrange the asparagus on the hot griddle. Cook for 1½ minutes, pushing down on top of the spears with the base of a clean heavy pan, so they steam as well as grill, and the spears will be crisp with a vibrant green colour. Turn the asparagus with a pair of tongs and replace the pan on top. Cook for a further 1½ minutes.

Slice the lamb and serve it with the asparagus and a good drizzle of salsa verde.

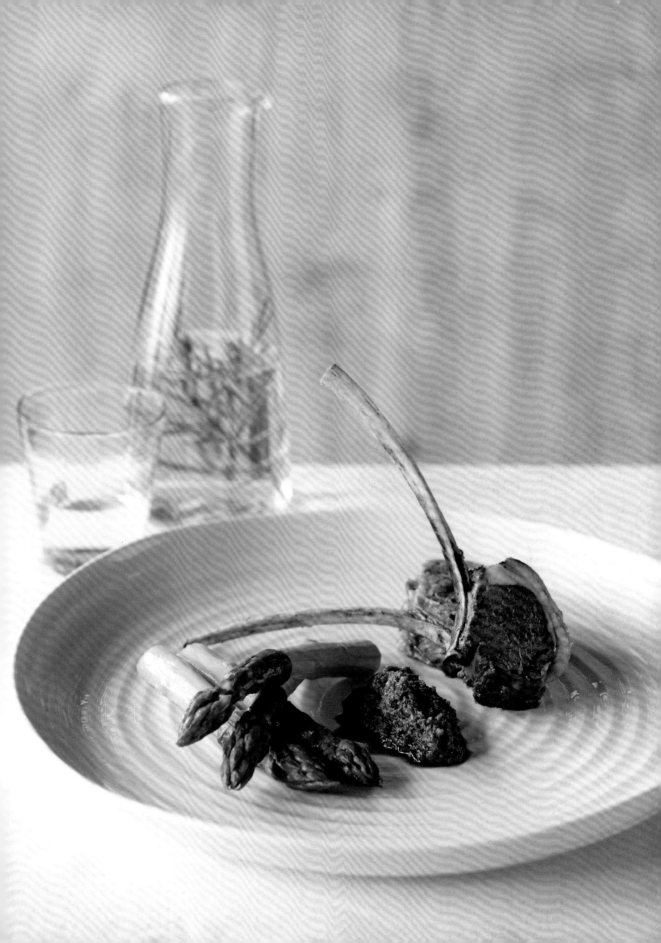

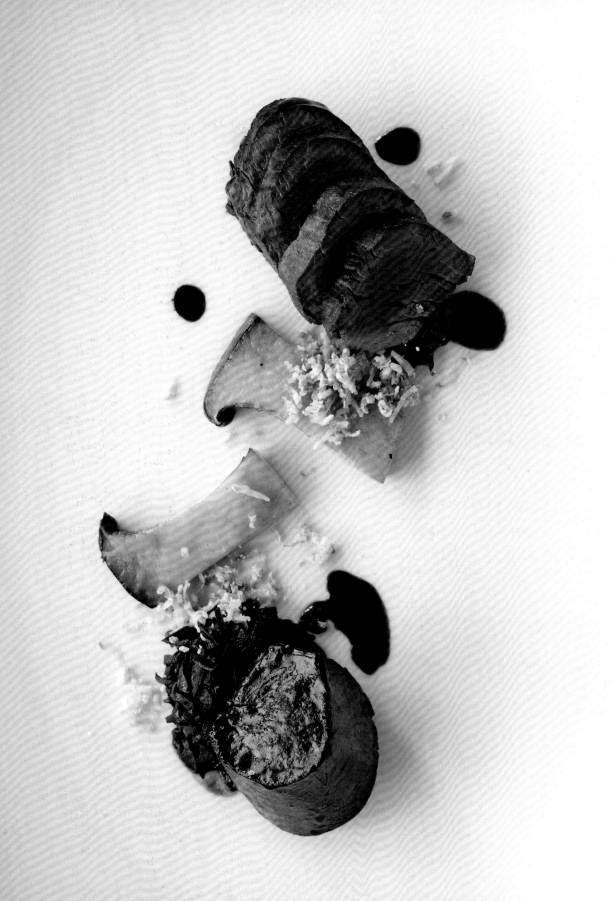

P Venison with red cabbage & sweet chestnut sauce

Venison is the leanest of all the red meats, but don't overcook or it will lose its tenderness. Searing the fillet seals in the juices and retains the flavour. This is an impressive dish for a dinner party as the tastes and textures complement each other beautifully.

Serves 4

300ml (½ pint/scant 1¼ cups) Chicken Broth (see page 44)

4 king oyster mushrooms

200g (7oz) vacuum-packed sweet chestnuts

4 juniper berries

knob of clarified butter

450g (1lb) venison loin, trimmed and sinews removed

salt and ground black pepper

10g (½oz) coconut oil

For the red cabbage:

300g (10oz) red cabbage, finely shredded

100ml (3½fl oz/generous ⅓ cup) cider vinegar

4 tsp maple syrup

75g (3oz) Braeburn apple, grated on a large grater

1 cinnamon stick

4 allspice berries

2 cloves

4 cardamom pods

2 bay leaves

Make the red cabbage: thinly slice it with a knife or a mandolin. Do not use the white root. Put all the ingredients in a stainless steel pan and bring to the boil. Cover with the lid, reduce the heat and cook gently for 40–50 minutes until tender. Add a little water halfway through if it seems dry and stir occasionally. Strain through a colander, reserve the cooking liquid which can be reduced to syrup and added to the chestnut sauce.

Bring the chicken broth to a simmer over a high heat. Cut the mushrooms in half and blanch them in the broth for 2 minutes. Remove with a slotted spoon and allow to cool ready for pan-frying later.

Reduce the broth by boiling to one-third of the original volume over a high heat, then add the reduced red cabbage syrup, half the chestnuts and the juniper berries. Cook for a further 10 minutes before adding a knob of butter and blending it with a stick blender until smooth. Pass through a sieve to make a rich gravy to serve with the venison.

Season the venison with salt and pepper. Heat a large frying pan and add the coconut oil. Sear the venison all over, then reduce the heat and pan-fry for a few minutes. Add a knob of butter and continue cooking, basting the venison from time to time, for about 8 minutes until cooked but still pink. Remove from the pan and set aside to rest for 15 minutes in a warm place.

In the same pan, sauté the blanched mushrooms for 2 minutes on each side until golden brown. Meanwhile, reheat the red cabbage. Slice the venison and arrange on serving plates with the mushrooms and the gravy. Grate the remaining sweet chestnuts over the top with a fine grater.

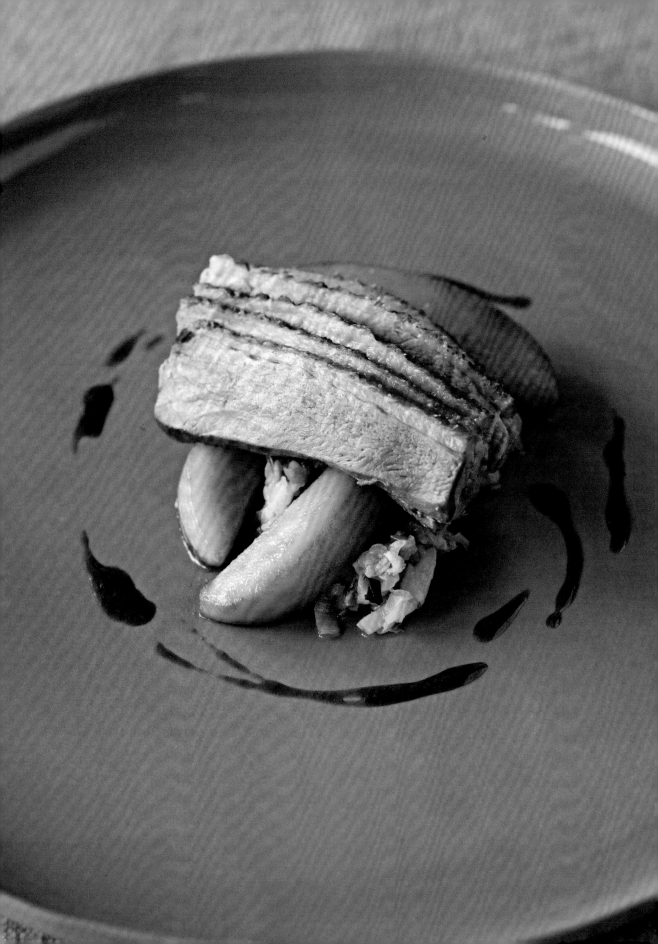

P Five-spiced duck with fermented cabbage & spiced pears

Sometimes you can include a fermented food in your main meal rather than eating sauerkraut or bitters beforehand. Duck is one of the richest poultry meats and the breasts are irresistible combined with sweet spiced pears and sour fermented cabbage in this mouthwatering dish.

Serves 4

4 small Barbary duck breasts

1 tbsp five-spice powder

2 Conference pears

2 cloves

1 star anise

3 allspice berries

1 tsp coriander seeds

50ml (2fl oz/scant ¼ cup) cider vinegar

50ml (2fl oz/scant ¼ cup) maple syrup

200ml (7fl oz/generous ¾ cup) Chicken Broth (see page 44)

50g (2oz/⅓ cup) frozen blackcurrants

sea salt

50g (2oz/½ stick) unsalted butter

120g (3¾oz) Thai fermented napa (see page 43)

Prepare the duck breasts by lightly scoring the skin with a sharp knife, then rub half of the five-spice powder into the skin and set aside until you're ready to cook them. Peel and core the pears and cut each one into 8 wedges.

Using a spice grinder or a pestle and mortar, grind the cloves, star anise, allspice and coriander seeds. In a small pan over a low heat, dry-toast the spices for a couple of minutes to release their natural oils, then add the cider vinegar. Increase the heat and cook until reduced by half, and then add the maple syrup, chicken broth and frozen blackcurrants.

Continue cooking until the mixture has reduced by half. Add the pear wedges and cook for 4–5 minutes, so they are partially cooked. Remove the pears to a plate and continue reducing the liquid down to a syrupy consistency, which can be passed through a fine sieve into a small bowl ready to finish later.

To cook the duck breasts, season them with sea salt on both sides. Place a frying pan over a medium heat and fry the duck, skin-side down, in the pan. Gradually turn up the heat to render all the fat from the duck – this takes about 10 minutes. When the skin is golden brown and crisp, turn the duck over and cook for 2 minutes on the other side. The breasts should be perfectly cooked. Remove from the heat and allow to rest.

To make the sauce, pour off any excess fat from the pan, add a little butter and the remaining five-spice powder, and pan-fry the poached pears on both sides until golden brown.

Warm the Thai fermented napa in a separate covered pan over a low heat for 2–3 minutes. To finish the sauce, add the syrupy reduction and warm over a low heat. Add the remaining butter.

Slice the duck breasts. Serve them with the warm Thai fermented napa and pears with a drizzle of the sauce.

NUTRITION FACTS

Duck provides B vitamins, zinc and Omega-3 and -6 to support immunity as well as being a rich source of protein for rebuilding and regenerating gut tissue.

(P) Sea bass with leeks, lemon & butternut squash purée

Sea bass is one of the best white fish – firm yet delicate and a superb choice for all palates. Pan-frying the leeks caramelizes them and enhances their depth of flavour. Do take care to brown, but not to burn, the skin of the sea bass as the beneficial essential fats lie just below it.

Serves 4

150ml (5fl oz/generous ½ cup) white wine

150ml (5fl oz/generous ½ cup) water

seeds of ½ vanilla pod (bean)

220g (7½oz) red and black seedless grapes

100ml (3½fl oz/generous ⅓ cup) fish stock

30g (1¼oz) softened unsalted butter

1 tsp toasted cumin seeds, ground

pinch of sea salt

1 tsp grated lemon zest

1 tsp lemon juice

200g (7oz) butternut squash, peeled, deseeded and finely diced

200ml (7fl oz/generous ¾ cup) Chicken Broth (see page 44)

20g (¾oz) preserved lemon, finely chopped

1 tsp local runny honey

ground black pepper

1 small leek, cut into 5mm (¼in) slices

10g (½oz) clarified butter

4 x 125g (4oz) sea bass fillets, boned and skinned

Bring the white wine and water to the boil in a pan set over a medium heat. Add the vanilla pod (bean) and seeds and simmer for 5 minutes. Add the grapes and gently simmer for 4 minutes.

Use a slotted spoon to remove the grapes from the liquid and place them on dehydrator trays. Dehydrate at 130°C, 266°F for 6 hours. Alternatively, put the poached grapes on a silicone-lined tray and dry them in a cool oven at 110°C, 225°F, Gas mark ¼ for 4 hours.

Reserve one-third of the white wine cooking liquor in the pan and add the fish stock. Cook it until reduced down to a syrup ready to make the sauce later.

Thoroughly mix together the softened butter with the cumin seeds, sea salt, lemon zest and juice.

Make the butternut squash purée: put the squash in a pan and cover with the chicken broth. Bring to the boil, then reduce the heat and cook until soft. Remove from the heat, drain and liquidize with the preserved lemon, honey and a knob of cumin butter. Season to taste with salt and pepper. (Do not use too much salt as the preserved lemons are quite salty.)

Pan-fry the leek over a low heat in a little of the clarified butter until golden brown on both sides.

Heat a large frying pan over a medium heat and fry the sea bass fillets, skin-side down, for 3 minutes in the remaining clarified butter. Turn them over and cook for 1 minute on the other side.

Gently warm the reduced sauce and add the remaining cumin butter, so it melts into the sauce. Add a squeeze of lemon juice. Serve the fish on top of a little sauce with the butternut purée. Put the warmed grapes and leeks on top.

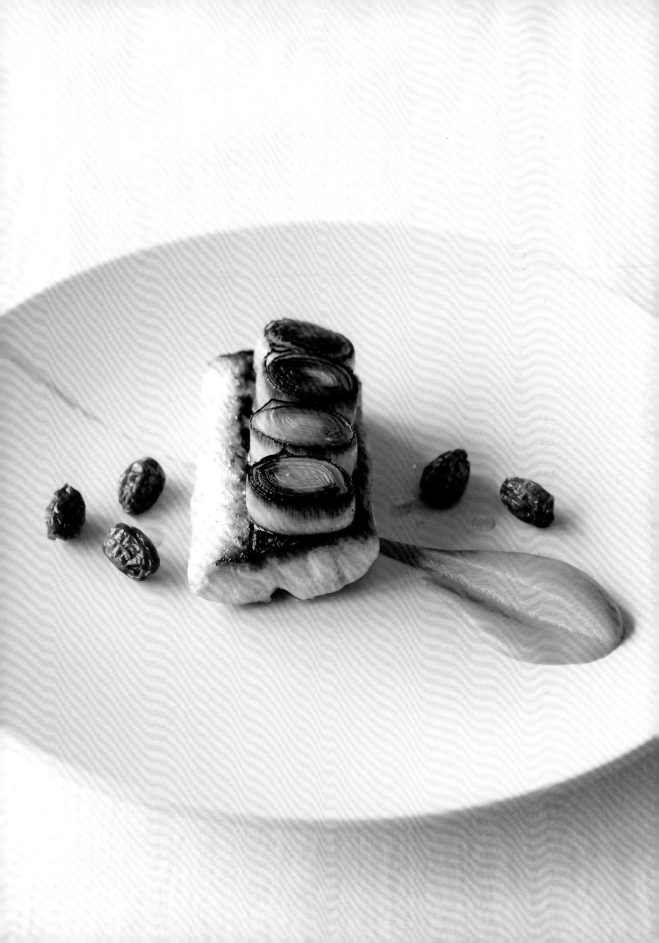

P Sea trout with pickled cucumber & tenderstem broccoli

Sea trout is sweeter and lighter than salmon and has a more delicate taste. Sorrel may be difficult to source but is well worth looking for – it may even grow wild in your own garden. Rich in antioxidants, beta-carotene and Vitamin C, it is a great flavour enhancer for soups and sauces.

Serves 4

1 cucumber

pinch of sea salt

4 tsp cider vinegar

1 tsp chopped dill

juice of ½ lemon

200g (7oz) tenderstem broccoli

30g (1¼oz/3 tbsp) clarified butter

20g (¾oz) sorrel

1 tsp coconut oil

4 x 125g (4oz) sea trout fillets, skin on, scaled and boned

To prepare the cucumber, peel away the outer skin with a potato peeler and then cut it in half lengthways. Remove and discard the seeds. Cut the outer part of the cucumber with a potato peeler or sharp knife into long ribbons ready to marinate.

Sprinkle the cucumber trimmings and seeds with the sea salt and place them in a colander with a bowl set underneath to collect the juice – you will only need about 50ml (2fl oz/scant ¼ cup). Add the cider vinegar, dill and lemon juice to the cucumber juice and then marinate the ribbons of cucumber for about 1 hour.

Trim the broccoli stalks halfway up, reserving the ends. Blanch the tops in boiling salted water for 1 minute, then refresh under cold running water. Shred the remaining stalks finely and sweat them in most of the butter in a small covered pan for about 15–20 minutes, until soft. Add the sorrel, season to taste with salt and pepper and then blend until smooth. Keep warm.

Heat a non-stick frying pan over a high heat and melt the coconut oil until smoking. Season the sea trout with salt and pepper and fry, skin-side down, for 3 minutes. Turn the sea trout over and fry for 1½ minutes on the other side until cooked.

Meanwhile, using the hot pan from cooking the sea trout, melt the remaining butter and reheat the blanched tenderstem broccoli tops. Serve the sea trout with the marinated cucumber, tenderstem purée and broccoli.

NUTRITION FACTS

Sea trout is rich in Omega-3 as it is a deep-water fish and not farmed in lakes or rivers. It is a good source of zinc and selenium, both required for a strong immune system, as well as vitamins B3, B6 and B12 which are needed for energy, clear thinking and concentration.

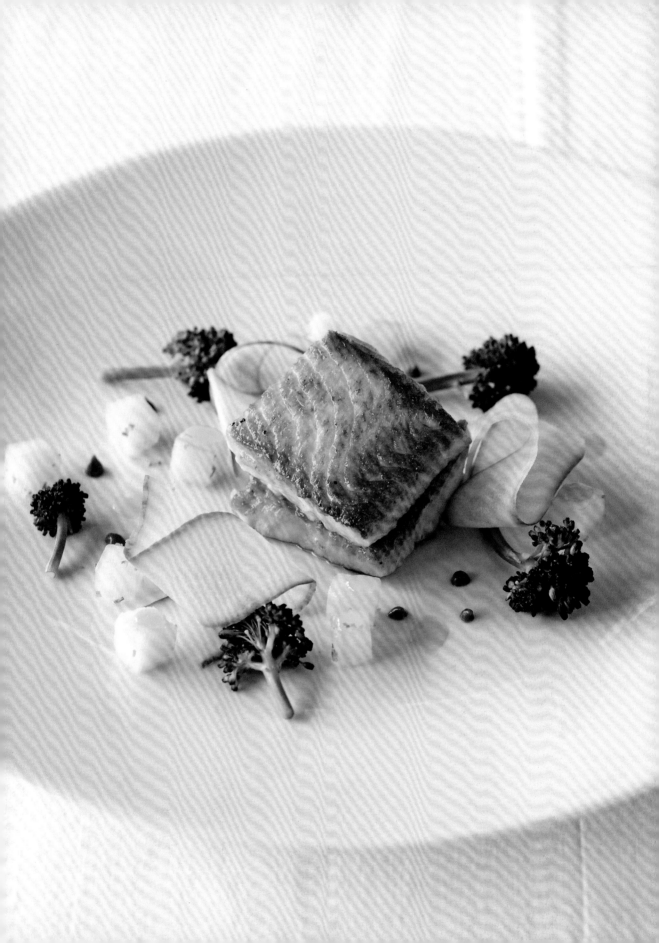

(P) Halibut with grey chanterelles, parsley root & blood orange

Source wild mushrooms carefully, as quality and freshness are tantamount to their flavour. Always handle them with care and, rather than washing them, gently rub away any dirt without bruising the fragile flesh. Their intense flavour perfectly complements the delicate sweetness of the halibut.

Serves 4

4 parsley roots (or parsnips if unavailable)

120ml (4fl oz/½ cup) Chicken Broth (see page 44)

50g (2oz/4 tbsp) clarified butter plus extra for cooking the parsley and fish

salt and ground black pepper

leaves from 4 thyme sprigs

4 x 125g (4oz) halibut fillets, boned and skinned

80g (3oz) grey chanterelles (or golden)

For the blood orange dressing:

4 blood oranges

1 star anise

½ tsp coriander seeds

50ml (2fl oz/scant ¼ cup) extra virgin olive oil

1 tsp lemon juice

Preheat the oven to 180°C, 350°F, Gas mark 4.

Peel the parsley roots with a potato peeler, then cut the tips into 5cm (2in) fine batons ready for roasting later. Chop the remaining parsley roots finely and place them in a small pan with the chicken broth. Cook over a medium heat until soft, then blend, using a hand blender, with the butter and salt and pepper until you have a smooth purée.

To make the blood orange dressing, juice 3 of the oranges into a small pan. Remove the segments from the other orange and set aside for the garnish. Add the star anise and coriander seeds to the orange juice in the pan. Reduce by cooking over a medium heat to about 3 tablespoons. Transfer to a jug or bowl and, using a hand blender, slowly blend in the olive oil to make an emulsion, then add the lemon juice.

Put the parsley roots with the thyme leaves and half the remaining butter in an ovenproof dish and roast in the preheated oven for 15 minutes until golden brown.

Heat some more butter over a high heat in a non-stick frying pan. Season the fish fillets and fry them on both sides for 1 minute before finishing in the oven for 4 minutes. Remove from the oven and keep warm on a plate.

Using the same pan, gently sauté the mushrooms over a medium heat with the remaining butter for 2 minutes.

Serve the fish on top of the roasted parsley roots with a smear of parsley purée and the reserved blood orange segments. Add a little dressing around the edge.

CHEF'S TIP

To give the dressing a really intense flavour, you must reduce the sauce significantly, stirring constantly.

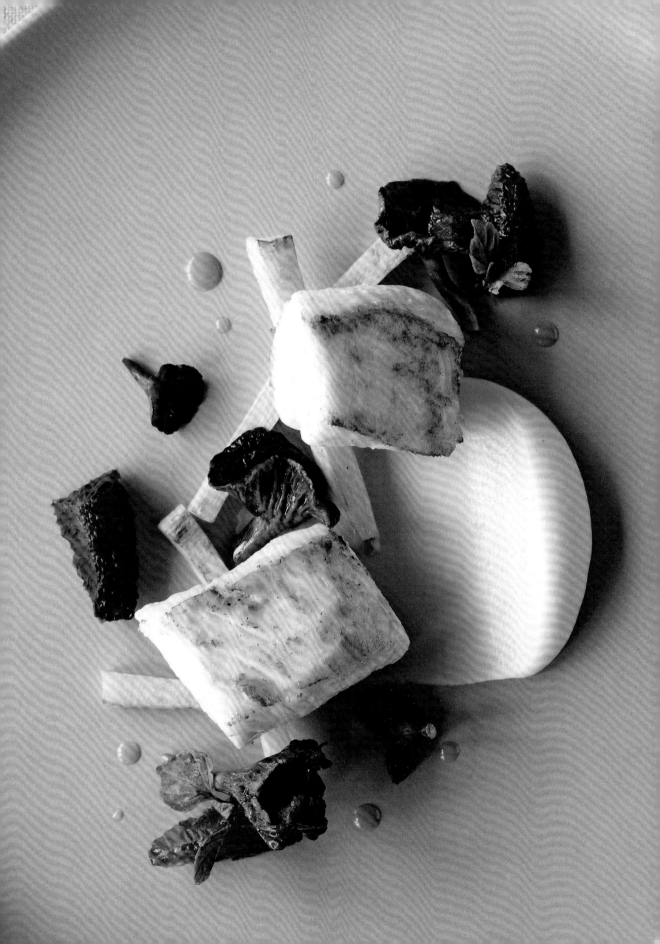

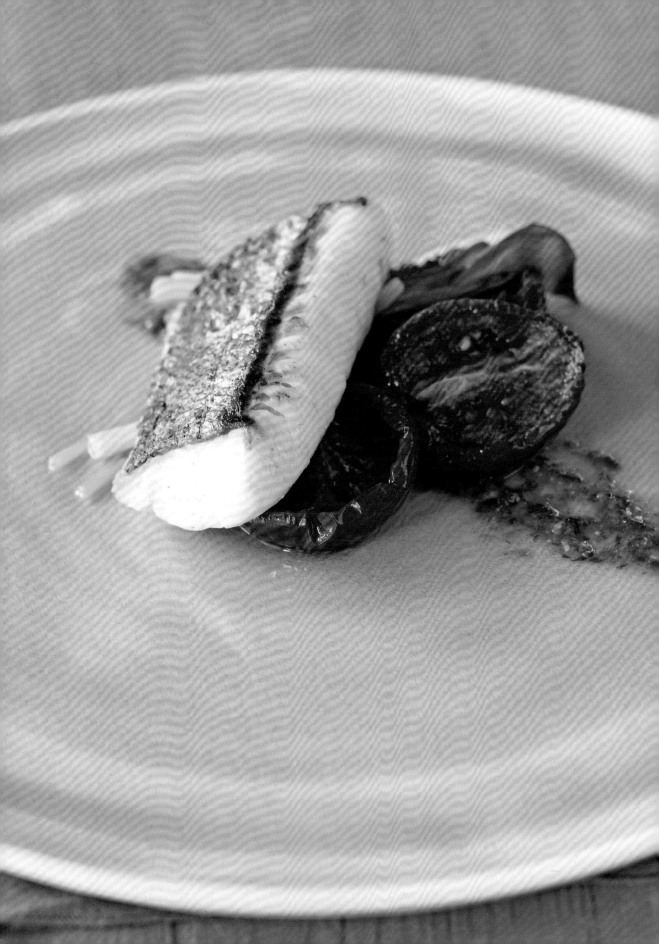

(P) Baked hake & tomatoes with garlic & hazelnut pesto

This pesto recipe is so versatile and is delicious served with roasted vegetables and salads. The quantities given below allow for more than this recipe, so try it with other vegetable dishes, too. You can keep the pesto fresh in a sealed jar in the fridge for several weeks.

Serves 4

300g (10oz) baby plum tomatoes

2 tbsp extra virgin olive oil

1 small bunch of lemon thyme, leaves removed from stalks

4 x 125g (4oz) hake (or white fish) fillets, skinned and boned

squeeze of lemon juice

2 large fat broccoli stalks from calabrese heads

5g (¼oz) coconut oil

For the garlic & hazelnut pesto:

100g (3½oz) wild garlic leaves, washed

100ml (3½fl oz/generous ⅓ cup) extra virgin olive oil

50g (2oz/⅓ cup) hazelnuts, roasted and skins, removed

50g (2oz/¼ cup) toasted pine nuts (pignoli)

juice of 1 lemon

1 tsp local runny honey

salt and ground black pepper

For the black garlic emulsion (optional):

150ml (¼ pint/⅔ cup) extra virgin olive oil

1 organic free-range egg yolk

6 black garlic cloves

2 tsp lemon juice

salt and ground black pepper

Preheat the oven to 130°C, 250°F, Gas mark ½.

To semi-dry the tomatoes, cut them in half, sprinkle with salt, and arrange them, cut-side up, on a non-stick baking sheet. Drizzle with the olive oil and rub with thyme. Cook in the preheated oven for 50–60 minutes until dehydrated slightly – this will intensify the flavour of the tomatoes and give them a lovely chewiness.

Make the pesto: remove the stalks from the wild garlic leaves and put into a food processor with the olive oil, hazelnuts, pine nut (pignoli), lemon juice, honey, salt and pepper and blitz until smooth. Spoon into a sterilized jar and keep in the fridge.

To make the black garlic emulsion (if using): simply whisk the oil gradually into the egg yolk, then blend in the other ingredients with a hand blender to make a smooth emulsion.

Increase the oven temperature to 200°C, 400°F, Gas mark 6.

Take a piece of aluminium foil large enough to fit all the pieces of hake within a single parcel. Spread the foil with a little of the pesto and place the hake on top. Season lightly with salt and pepper and a squeeze of lemon juice. Fold the foil over the fish and seal the edges tightly. Place on a baking sheet and cook in the preheated oven for 15 minutes until the fish is cooked.

Meanwhile, square off the edges of the broccoli stalks and cut them into thin 2mm (⅛in) x 6cm (2in) strips. Heat a frying pan over a high heat, and stir-fry the broccoli strips in a little coconut oil for 1½ minutes. Season with salt and pepper.

Arrange the tomato and broccoli stalks on the serving plates. Place the hake on top and drizzle with a little pesto. Serve with the black garlic emulsion (if using).

Post-Plan special occasions

Once you have completed the Plan, the additional permitted ingredients, including some grains, cheeses and root vegetables, allow you to expand your repertoire. The following recipes include Jerusalem artichokes, butter (lima) beans, quinoa, parsnips, and rye flakes. However, the emphasis still remains on the core animal proteins and vegetable accompaniments.

P+ Pan-fried flat-iron steak with shallots & jerusalem artichokes

Jerusalem artichokes are not eaten often yet they have an exquisite taste when roasted simply with butter and lemon juice. The richness of the Savoy cabbage, which is blanched and then pan-fried, coupled with the Port-drenched shallots is the perfect complement to the steak.

Serves 4

200g (7oz) Jerusalem artichokes

5g (¼oz/1 tsp) butter

1 tsp lemon juice

8 banana shallots, peeled and cut in half lengthways

150ml (5fl oz/scant ⅔ cup) Port

250ml (8fl oz/1 cup) Chicken Broth (see page 44)

20g (¾oz) mustard seeds

40ml (1½fl oz/3 tbsp) water

40ml (1½fl oz/3 tbsp) cider vinegar

4 tsp local runny honey

pinch of salt

30g (1¼oz) Savoy cabbage

4 x 125g (4oz) flat-iron steaks

ground black pepper

20g (¾oz/1½ tbsp) clarified butter

Preheat the oven to 180°C, 350°F, Gas mark 4.

Make a foil parcel and add the artichokes, butter and lemon juice. Seal the parcel, then bake in the preheated oven for 45 minutes. Peel the artichokes and cut them into 5mm (¼in) slices. Set aside.

Place the shallots, flat-side down, in a frying pan with the Port and chicken broth and reduce over a medium heat until nearly all the stock has been absorbed and the shallots are soft and sticky. Reserve a little of the reduction to brush over the steaks later.

Soak the mustard seeds in hot water for 10 minutes. Drain and then add the cider vinegar, honey and salt. Stir to cover the mustard seeds, then leave for at least 30 minutes until they plump up and absorb the vinegar.

Blanch the Savoy cabbage in a pan of boiling water for 2 minutes. Refresh under cold running water and then drain.

Heat a frying pan over a high heat. Season the steaks with salt and pepper and fry them in the clarified butter for 2–3 minutes on each side, according to taste. Remove from the pan and rest in a warm place for 5 minutes.

Using the same pan, fry the artichokes until golden brown, then remove and add the cabbage. Stir-fry with a little salt and pepper for just long enough to warm everything through.

Brush the steaks with the reserved glaze and serve with the cabbage, artichokes, glazed shallots and pickled mustard seeds.

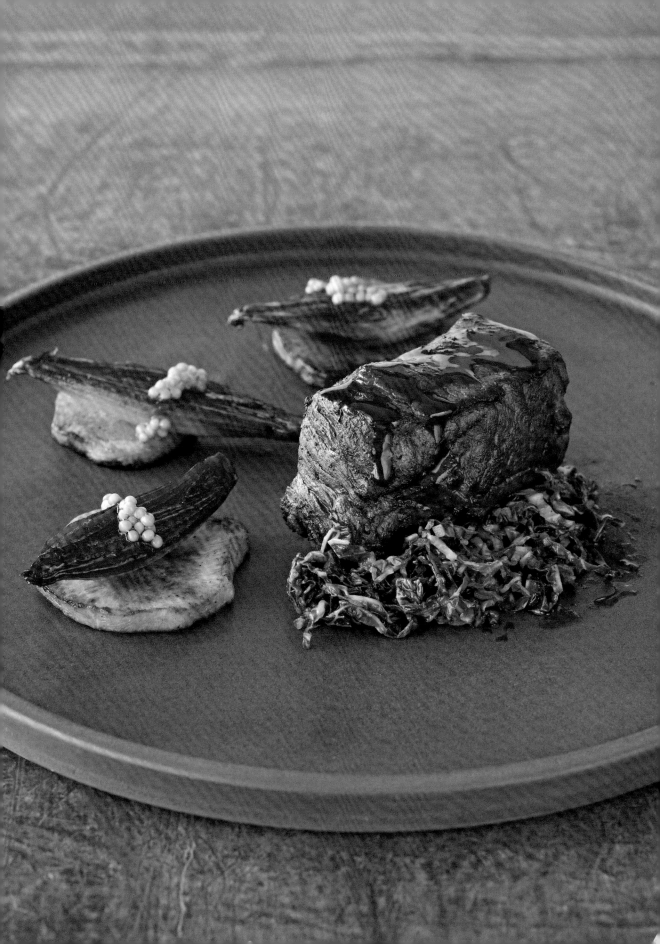

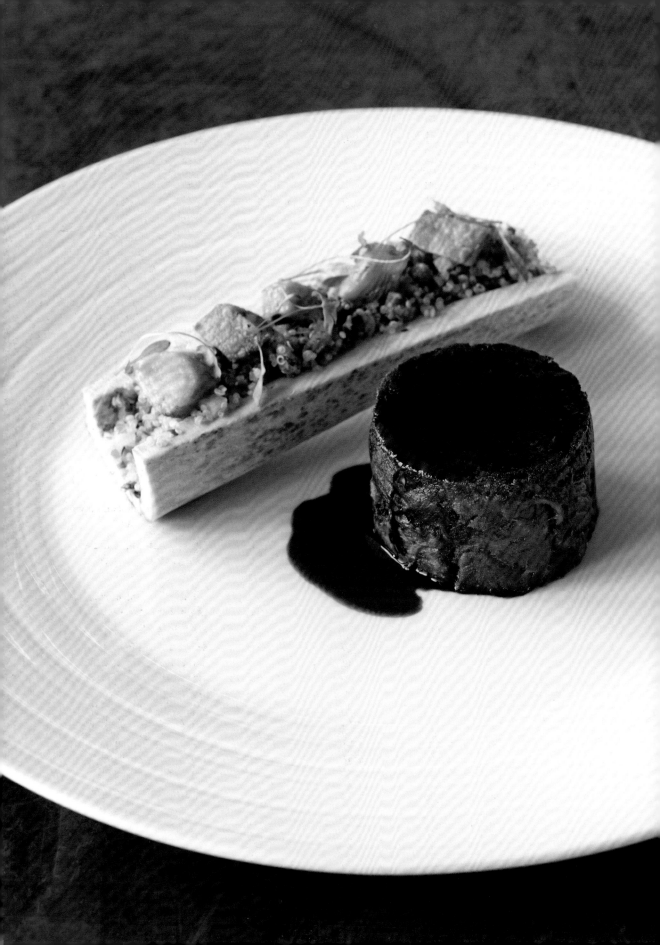

P+ Braised shin of beef, bone marrow & horseradish quinoa

Shin of beef has become less popular as most of us opt for easier cuts, yet this is a really tasty and nutrient-rich dish, which adheres to the beauty of the Slow Food Movement. The meat is cooked at a very low temperature for several hours, preserving the nutrients and intensifying the flavour.

Serves 4

2 tbsp clarified butter

2 carrots, finely chopped

2 celery sticks, finely chopped

1 onion, finely chopped

1 garlic bulb, cut in half

1kg (2lb 3½oz) shin of beef

chicken stock or water to cover

100ml (3½fl oz/generous ⅓ cup) Madeira

4 bay leaves

20 black peppercorns

1 bunch of fresh thyme

For the quinoa:

40g (1½oz/scant ¼ cup) quinoa

20g (¾oz) carrot, chopped

20g (¾oz) celeriac, chopped

15g (½oz) shallot, chopped

leaves stripped from a few thyme sprigs

2 tbsp clarified butter

½ tsp grated fresh horseradish

1 tbsp mixed chopped parsley, chervil and chives

Heat the clarified butter in a pan and add the carrot, celery, onion and garlic and fry until it starts to colour. Transfer to a heatproof casserole pot and add the beef. Cover with the stock or water, and add the Madeira, bay leaves and peppercorns. Cover with a lid and cook over a very low heat at a bare simmer for 3 hours.

After 3 hours, check that the beef is cooked (it should gently break apart with ease). Remove from the stock and set aside to cool for 10 minutes. Gently remove the connective tissue and any sinew from the beef and set the meat aside. Roll out a sheet of cling film (plastic wrap) and place the beef at one edge. Roll into a sausage shape 5cm (2in) thick, then tie both ends and leave in the fridge to set.

Strain the stock into a clean pan and reduce over a medium heat until it's one-quarter of its original volume (this will be the final sauce).

Preheat the oven to 170°C, 325°F, Gas mark 3.

Put the quinoa in a pan and cover with twice its volume of water. Simmer gently for 20 minutes.

Meanwhile, in a clean pan sauté the carrot, celeriac, shallot and thyme in 1 tablespoon of the clarified butter until lightly coloured.

Place the marrow bones on a shallow baking tray and roast in the preheated oven for 15 minutes. With a spoon, scoop out the bone marrow and reserve until later.

When the quinoa is cooked, strain it and add the cooked vegetables, horseradish and chopped herbs. Mix together and spoon back into the bones, placing pieces of the cooked bone marrow on top.

Take the beef out of the fridge and remove the cling film (plastic wrap). Cut into 4 portions. Heat 1 tbsp butter in a frying pan and cook the beef portions, flat-side down, over a medium to high heat for 3 minutes. Add 4 tablespoons of the sauce and turn the heat down to low. Cook for 5 minutes turning the beef halfway through the cooking time. Pop into the oven for 10 minutes to warm through.

Serve each portion of beef on a serving plate with the bone filled with quinoa and vegetables, and drizzle with the remaining sauce.

P+ Pan-fried calves' liver with butter bean & sage purée, black pudding bonbons and green beans

Calves' liver is the sweetest and gentlest flesh of all offal but you must take care not to over-cook it. The butter (lima) bean and sage purée provides a creamier alternative to traditional mashed potato. The black pudding bonbons are an optional extra but well worth the time they take to make.

Serves 4

150g (5oz) dried butter (lima) beans, soaked overnight in water with added lemon juice

20g (¾oz/1½ tbsp) butter

8 sage leaves

3 rashers pancetta (see page 69), chopped

20g (¾oz) shallots, finely chopped

25g (1oz/2 tbsp) clarified butter, plus extra for shallow-frying

100g (3½oz) black pudding, broken into pieces

20g (¾oz) white quinoa, ground into flour

150g (5oz) fine green beans, trimmed

400g (14oz) calves' liver, thinly sliced

Drain the butter (lima) beans and cook in a pan of simmering water for 45 minutes. Drain and set aside.

Heat the butter in a small pan over a medium heat and fry the sage leaves without browning. Add 4 sage leaves to the butter (lima) beans and, using a stick blender, bend to a smooth purée. Add a little water if necessary to get the right consistency for smearing the plates. Reserve the remaining sage leaves for the garnish.

Fry the pancetta and shallots in the clarified butter until golden brown. Add to the black pudding and blend together using a stick blender. Roll the mixture into 8 balls and coat them lightly with the quinoa flour. Shallow-fry them in a little clarified butter, turning occasionally, until crisp on the outside.

Blanch the green beans in a pan of boiling water for 4 minutes. Drain well.

Heat a frying pan over a high heat, add the remaining clarified butter and fry the calves' liver quickly for 1 minute on each side.

Serve the calves' liver, topped with the fried sage leaves, with the black pudding bonbons, butter (lima) bean and sage purée and the green beans.

NUTRITION FACTS

Calves' liver provides one of the richest sources of iron known to man and it is therefore hugely beneficial to health, especially if you engage in active sports.

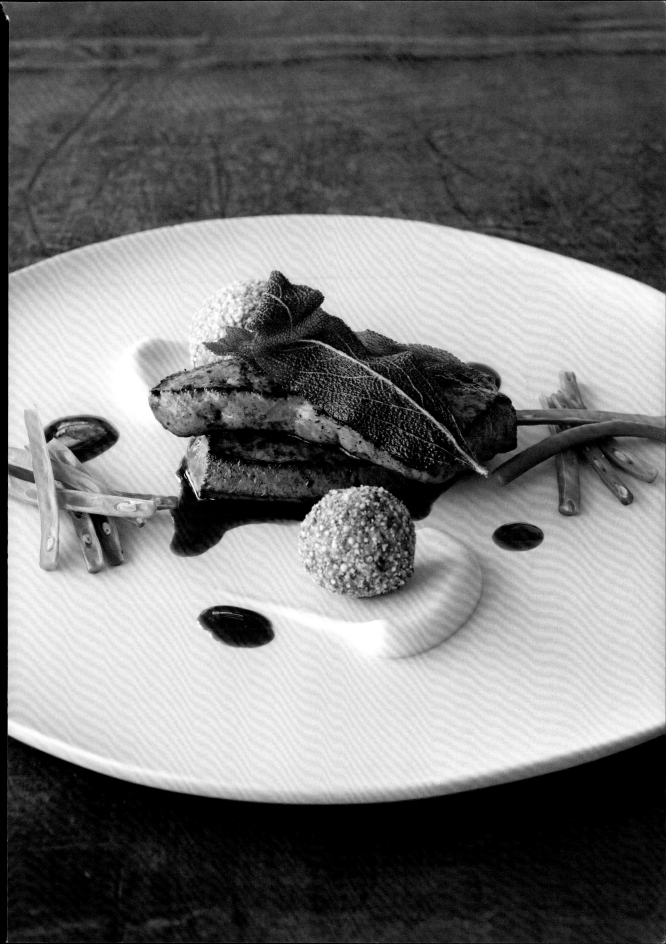

P+ Guinea fowl ballotine with orange-glazed belgian endive

Guinea fowl is very tasty and surpasses chicken by a mile for flavour and texture. The bitterness of the chicory (Belgian endive) is reduced by soaking and pan-frying it with orange juice, and balanced by the sweetness of the root vegetables. The toasted rye flakes complete this dish.

Serves 6

150g (5oz) sea salt crystals

4 large carrots, washed but not peeled

2 heads chicory (Belgian endive)

20g (¾oz/1 tbsp) butter

200ml (7fl oz/generous ¾ cup) orange juice

4 x 125g (4oz) guinea fowl breasts

40g (1½oz/3 tbsp) clarified butter

20g (¾oz) rye flakes

pinch of Tangerine, cumin, fennel & chipotle salt (see page 36), plus additional salt for sprinkling

Preheat the oven to 180°C, 350°F, Gas mark 4.

Sprinkle the sea salt crystals over a baking tray. Arrange the carrots on top and bake in the preheated oven for 50 minutes until softened. Remove the carrots, then shake off the salt and peel them with a small knife before cutting each carrot in half lengthways.

Cut each chicory (Belgian endive) head in half and soak for 10 minutes in cold water to remove any bitterness. Place the chicory (Belgian endive), flat-side down, in a shallow pan with the butter and cook over a low heat for 5 minutes. Add the orange juice and cook over a medium heat until reduced to a glaze.

To make the ballotines, roll each individual guinea fowl breast in a layer of cling film (plastic wrap) into a sausage shape. Wrap in another layer of cling film (plastic wrap) and then put the ballotines into a small deep pan. Cover with cold water, bring to the boil, then reduce the heat and simmer for 4 minutes.

Remove the ballotines from the pan and take off the layers of cling film (plastic wrap). Heat a large frying pan over a medium heat and brown the ballotines for a couple of minutes in some of the clarified butter, turning them occasionally until browned all over. Remove from the pan and roast in the preheated oven for 5 minutes. Remove and set aside to rest for 5 minutes, reserving the cooking juices.

Put the remaining clarified butter in a pan with the rye flakes and flavoured salt. Slowly heat over a low heat until gently toasted.

To serve, warm the baked carrots in the cooking juices from the ballotines. Slice the ballotines in half and then arrange them on serving plates with the glazed chicory (Belgian endive), carrots and a sprinkling of the toasted rye. Lightly season the ballotines with a little flavoured salt.

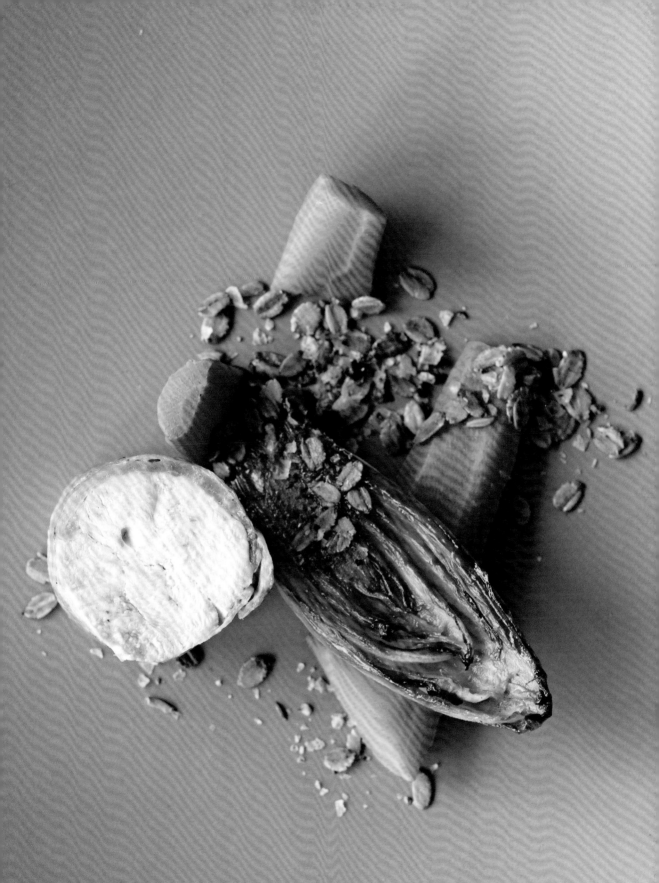

P+ King scallops with cauliflower, anchovy emulsion & vierge dressing

Vierge dressing is for people who love hollandaise sauce but prefer something lighter. King scallops are the ultimate in seafood, but you must source good-quality fresh ones. The beauty of this dish is its simplicity: you can prepare the emulsion and dressing in advance and store them in the fridge until needed.

Serves 4

1 small cauliflower

20g (¾oz/1½ tbsp) unsalted butter

1 tsp clarified butter

12 king scallops

For the anchovy emulsion:

40g (1½oz) anchovies in brine

15g (½oz) capers

1 tbsp olive oil

½ tsp Dijon mustard

1 tsp water

For the vierge dressing:

1 tbsp olive oil

1 tsp cider vinegar

½ tsp Dijon mustard

15g (½oz) shallot, finely diced

1 plum tomato, skinned, deseeded and cut into 5mm (¼in) dice

1 slice of garlic

1 tsp chopped chervil

salt and ground black pepper

Trim the cauliflower, divide into florets and cut into 5mm (¼in) slices. Bring a pan of water to the boil and blanch the cauliflower for 1 minute. Remove with a slotted spoon and refresh in cold water.

Make the anchovy emulsion: put all the ingredients in a jug blender and blend together until puréed.

To make the vierge dressing, whisk together the olive oil, cider vinegar and Dijon mustard. Then add the shallot, tomato, garlic and herbs, and season to taste with salt and pepper.

In a frying pan set over a medium heat, melt the butter and then add the cauliflower slices. Cook for 4 minutes until they start to colour.

In a separate pan over a high heat, add the clarified butter and then the king scallops. Cook for 1½ minutes, then turn them over and cook for 30 seconds on the other side. Remove from the pan and leave to rest.

Arrange the scallops on top of the cauliflower. Drizzle the vierge dressing over the top and then add a few dots of the anchovy emulsion to the plates to serve.

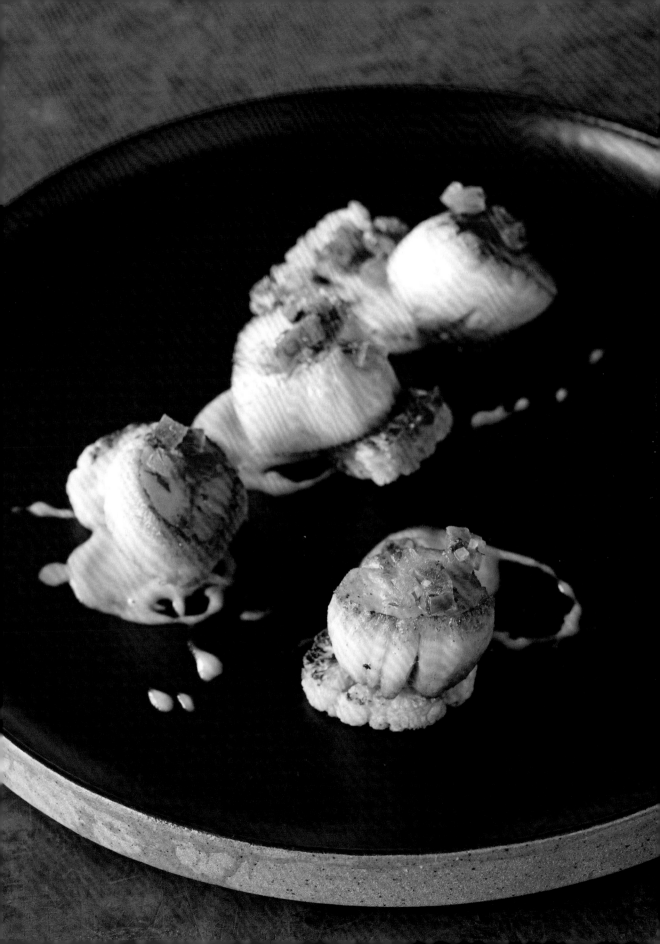

Suppliers

UK

NUTRITIONAL SUPPLEMENTS

Viridien
Digestive bitters.
www.viridien.com

Optibac
Probiotics.
www.optibac.com

Biokult
Probiotics.
www.biokult.com

Organic Burst
Superfoods – maca, spirulina,
chlorella powders.
www.organicburst.com

FOODS

The Chia Company
Chia seeds.
www.thechiaco.com.au

Premier Seeds
Seeds for sprouting.
www.premierseedsdirect.com

Mushroom Table
Mushrooms to buy, and foraging tours.
www.mushroomtable.com

The Real Food Company
Fermented foods.
www.realfoodcompany.com

The Real Food Store
Online company for organic coconut
oil, specialist superfoods and powders.
www.realfoodstore.co.uk

Biona
Online company for organic produce
of all types.
www.biona.com

Excalibur
Dehydrators.
www.amazon.com

RAW HONEY

Look for local beekeepers who sell
direct to the public.

US

Bob's Red Mill Natural Foods
Flour and grains.
www.bobsredmill.com

Whole Foods Market
Online company for organic produce
of all types.
www.wholefoodsmarket.com

**Frontier Natural products Co-op
and Simply Organic**
Natural and organic products –
herbs, spices and extracts.
www.frontiercoop.com

Navitas Naturals
Superfoods – minimally processed,
gluten-free and kosher.
www.navitasnaturals.com

Trader Joe's
Online company for organic and
all-natural produce.
www.traderjoes.com

US & AUSTRALIA

The Chia Company
Chia seeds.
www.thechiaco.com.au

Pukka Herbs
Organic herbs.
www.pukkaherbs.com

Acknowledgements

All good concepts are born out of sound philosophy, and time-tested,
medically-based concepts form the basis of this book.

Our sincere thanks go to Elaine Williams and Stephanie Moore, who
developed the outline of the Regime for Grayshott Spa. We have adapted
their recommendations to provide a sustainable 'at-home' Plan.

For Chris and his Team in the kitchen, who worked tirelessly, and
unselfishly, to develop realistic 'at-home' recipes, and to ensure that we
ignite the potential chef in every reader!

To Adam's wife Sonia, and son Woody, who dared to try the recipes in
the first place, and to Carrie for her devoted rendition from the kitchen
to the page.

To Jacqui Small, Heather Thomas and Maggie Town for their
unerring commitment to this beautiful book. To Lisa Linder for bringing
the recipes alive. To Fritha Saunders for coordinating this project. And to
Eleni Thoma, who supported Vicki throughout countless edits.

And to Simon Lowe, the owner of Grayshott Spa, who had the
foresight to understand that it takes many ingredients to make a delicious
dish, and for bringing us all together.

These are all the people it takes to produce a book of such
magnitude. We both thank you.

Adam and Vicki

Laptops
For Seniors
FOR
DUMMIES®

by Nancy Muir

WILEY

Laptops For Seniors For Dummies®

Published by
Wiley Publishing, Inc.
111 River Street
Hoboken, NJ 07030-5774

www.wiley.com

Copyright © 2010 by Wiley Publishing, Inc., Indianapolis, Indiana

Published by Wiley Publishing, Inc., Indianapolis, Indiana

Published simultaneously in Canada

For general information on our other products and services, please contact our Customer Care Department within the U.S. at 877-762-2974, outside the U.S. at 317-572-3993, or fax 317-572-4002.

For technical support, please visit www.wiley.com/techsupport.

Wiley also publishes its books in a variety of electronic formats. Some content that appears in print may not be available in electronic books.

Library of Congress Control Number: 2010921233

ISBN: 978-0-470-57830-8

Manufactured in the United States of America

10 9 8 7 6 5 4 3 2 1

WILEY